To the living memory of my father, Dr. Harry L. Goldwag

Oh, heart, if the ignorant say to you that the soul perishes like the body, answer that the flower perishes but the seeds remain. This is the law of God.

—Kahlil Gibran

A human being is a part of the whole, called by us "universe," a part limited in time and space. He experiences himself, his thoughts and feelings, as something separate from the rest—a kind of optical delusion of his consciousness. This delusion is a kind of prison for us, restricting us to our personal decisions and to affection for a few persons nearest to us. Our task must be to free ourselves from this prison by widening our circle of compassion to embrace all living creatures and the whole nature in its beauty.

Albert Einstein

Elliott M. Goldwag, ed.
INNER BALANCE
The Power of Holistic Healing

Insights of Hans Selye,
Elisabeth Kübler-Ross,
Marcus Bach, and others

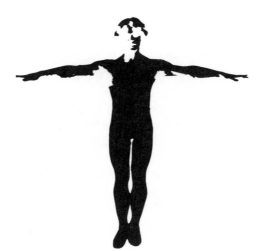

PRENTICE-HALL, INC., Englewood Cliffs, New Jersey 07632

Library of Congress Cataloging in Publication Data

Main entry under title:

Inner balance.

   (A Spectrum Book)
   Bibliography: p.
   Includes index.
   1.   Medicine—Philosophy.   2.   Mind and body.
3.   Medicine and religion.   4.   Health.   5.   Stress
(physiology)   6.   Holism.   I.   Goldwag, Elliott M.
R723.I56   615   79-14525
ISBN 0-13-465609-1
ISBN 0-13-465591-5 pbk.

A SPECTRUM BOOK

Editorial/production supervision by Shirley Covington
Manufacturing buyer: Cathie Lenard

10 9 8 7 6 5 4 3 2 1

Printed in the United States of America

PRENTICE-HALL INTERNATIONAL, INC., *London*
PRENTICE-HALL OF AUSTRALIA PTY. LIMITED, *Sydney*
PRENTICE-HALL OF CANADA, LTD., *Toronto*
PRENTICE-HALL OF INDIA, PRIVATE LIMITED, *New Delhi*
PRENTICE-HALL OF JAPAN, INC., *Tokyo*
PRENTICE-HALL OF SOUTHEAST ASIA PTE. LTD., *Singapore*
WHITEHALL BOOKS LIMITED, WELLINGTON, *New Zealand*

Contents

MALCOLM TODD

v

Preface

This book rises out of my conviction that the health care system is on the brink of an exciting rebirth. Through the work of thousands of researchers and practitioners, we are about to rediscover the thrilling truth of the meaning of healing: first, because the present methods of understanding and treating illness are proving to be counterproductive to the long-term health of individuals, and second, because new ideas about the cause of illness and its prevention promise a dramatic lowering of health costs.

This book highlights, through chapters written by thoughtful professionals in the health care system, that a better approach to healing can be achieved through methods of controlling the stress response. We can cope with our lives in a more beneficial way—a way that minimizes the damaging effects of stress while maximizing its positive aspects.

The means of dealing with stress is a matter of self-direction, using the power of our inner resources to maintain states of harmony and balance and thus producing greater self-fulfillment in our lives.

The philosophy and principles of this book establish a solid framework for what areas need to be explored and researched to maintain the health of our populations and to prevent illness from occurring.

My opinion is that disease and illness are abnormal, no matter what large numbers in our society are so affected. The words dis-order, dis-ease, dis-stress clearly indicate a deviation from the normal functioning of nature and of all living things—harmony and balance. Alterations from this state produce aberrations that result in symptoms and disease. It is my conviction that somewhere in the belief system of each person lie the self-limiting thoughts, distorted ideas, negative self-images, or other programmed attitudes that have produced alterations and disrupted or interfered with the balanced activity of normal functioning. Intimately involved in such belief systems is our relationship to our spiritual or God-self, which has become disturbed in some way that prevents our sharing the enormous source of strength available to us.

Many definititions of health have been offered in various types of literature, depending upon the perspective of the individual writer. One thing generally agreed upon, however, is that health is more than the absence of disease or illness—that it includes a fully productive, self-realized, expanded life of joy, happiness, and love in and for whatever one is doing. Each of us has a far greater role to play in the genesis of our illness or health than we have been willing to recognize or accept.

The idea for this book evolved from two unusual health conferences held in Houston, Texas in 1977 and 1978, where a number of the contributors gathered to present their ideas related to the future of health care in the United States. Together in one room were physicians, nurses, social workers, clergymen, psychologists, dentists, and nonprofessional people who were searching for better answers to the health problems we face as a nation. Though differing in professional backgrounds, everyone seemed to join together in a spirit of sharing ideas with one another and of gaining a better appreciation of each other, not as professionals, but as human beings.

It was a personal reward for me to organize these conferences and to enjoy the friendship of the dedicated participants. These meetings proved that there are physicians and other professionals in the health care system who are questioning some of the current practices and who are seeking better ways to improve the services they render and to enrich the quality of their lives. They were receptive to new thoughts and ideas that at times differed from what they had been taught.

The themes of both conferences focused on one predominant point: We have far greater control and direction over our lives and our health than we have believed we have. The same power that produces the altered state of illness is available to reproduce the state of health.

It seems to me that scientists are always exchanging ideas and writing papers directed to each other, but there doesn't seem to be enough exchange between all of us as human beings, both professionals and lay persons. I believe there is a great need for communication among us learning to speak the same language. This book is an expression of that need.

Some of us assume fragmented identities, one part scientist or professional, one part father or mother, another part friend, and another part churchgoer or spiritual person. Can we so easily compartmentalize our beliefs in each of these roles? Is it natural for us to be an eternal being on a day of worship but something else in our office or work?

This book is an attempt to contribute toward greater understanding by speaking largely in a nontechnical language about health care and thus offering the rich experience of these dedicated professionals to help people help themselves. We have attempted to minimize footnotes but have provided bibliographical references for further exploration. Each contributor has written an original paper for the book.

If you are a person suffering from a chronic disorder or have someone in your family who is so incapacitated, if you are in the helping profession as a practitioner or as a student, or if you are just someone interested in keeping yourself and your family healthy, you will find some provocative thoughts expressed by these experienced professionals that may help you.

Choices must always be made in this kind of ambitious undertaking. We have chosen to dip into many fields. A specialist in any one of these fields might be critical of the abbreviated treatment given to the subject in which he or she may have devoted the major part of his or her career. It is intended, however, that this book briefly synthesize many ideas. For those readers interested in a more in-depth study of any one subject, selections from the references and suggested readings should satisfy their need.

We do not suggest that you should avoid consulting a competent physician if you are ill. On the contrary, a physician is trained to understand the disease process and pathology and through this understanding and knowledge is able to isolate many variables and help guide you to a better understanding of what needs to be done to improve your health. This has been his traditional role since the time of Hippocrates; he is a guide, a teacher who works with the natural healing forces to help people heal themselves. The health care system is to help you help yourself stay healthy or get well and stay that way.

Dr. Malcolm Todd's introduction is particularly noteworthy in view of the prestigious position he held in the American Medical Association as its president in 1975. His emphasis on prevention of illness as the great challenge to modern medicine and his recognition that alternatives need to be examined in a responsible manner attest to the breadth of his vision and support his important leadership in organized medicine.

I believe that the contribution of Dr. Hans Selye to medicine is as momentous as Pasteur's germ theory of disease; the full implications of his work have still not been realized. Dr. Selye's careful and painstaking research of more than forty years to document scientifically the effect of stress on the biochemistry and physiology of the human organism is worthy of no less than the highest praise and recognition by the world of medicine and science.

In his first chapter, Dr. Selye briefly outlines and summarizes his monumental work on how stress affects human functioning and is the basis of disease. His second chapter highlights stress as a response that is individual to each person because of the way he or she perceives the world. The process of self-regulation is the means by which each of us can use stress to cope better and to change our responses to healthier adaptations. Dr. Selye's fame as one of the most respected researchers in scientific medicine lends particular emphasis to these points.

Dr. Charles Stroebel's experience as a physician and physiologist brings a rich combination of talent to discuss the field of autogenic training, or the means by which biofeedback and other self-directing exercises can actually teach people to change many symptoms and to alter the autonomic states of the body. The use of this training for providing self-help is growing at a rapid rate.

In the past ten years, meditation has become a popular subject in the United States. Various forms are proposed by different gurus, teachers, and masters to produce relaxed states or more peaceful, harmonious states of being. Dr. Syed Abdullah's experience in using forms of meditation combined with his clinical work provides us with the richness of the contribution of meditation in relieving many symptoms and helping improve the quality of one's life through inner harmony and guidance.

What has come to be recognized as groundbreaking work in a new way to look at helping patients overcome their cancer has been developed by Dr. Carl Simonton and his wife Stephanie Matthews–Simonton. Dr. Simonton is a recognized and respected oncologist (cancer specialist). He uses the accepted methods of treating cancer but has added the important dimensions of visual imagery and psychotherapy in helping patients who are willing to assume a role in their recovery to understand how they can reverse the cancer process.

Dr. Gerald Jampolsky has been working with children who suffer from catastrophic disorders like leukemia. Using guided imagery and a system of thought called spiritual psychotherapy, he has achieved remarkable results in reducing the fear, anxiety, and worry that are part of the unhappy circumstances surrounding a child's day-to-day world. Even though some children do not recover from their illness, the peaceful and meaningful growth achieved by these children and their families through the elimination of fear is most profound. Dr. Jampolsky's work is recognized throughout the nation as a major contribution toward helping children help themselves through self-direction.

There are many books on nutrition written by a wide variety of authors, some of whom have questionable credentials. The result is a great deal of confusion, which my brother, Dr. William Goldwag, seeks to dispel. His novel approach of relating nutrition not only to food but also to nourishment of the whole person reflects his own experience over many years in the practice of preventive medicine. His articles appear in a number of magazines and newspapers throughout the United States.

Recognizing the extraordinary power of spiritual thought in the health of the whole man, Dr. Marcus Bach shares his study of world religions and his personal experience in living with people representing these thoughts. He finds the common denominators that connect all religious thought and finds the means by which they are integrated into a developed medical model of health and wholeness.

Julian Byrd served as a hospital chaplain for many years, accumulating vast experiences both in his personal growth and with those he has counseled. His very human and compassionate understanding of the fear and anxiety of patients and their families enables him to relate his personal philosophy and to give examples of how spiritual help has enabled people to grow, recover faster, or die with dignity and in peace.

There has been a growing awareness among many therapists and counselors that the area of spiritual psychotherapy is most basic to the greater understanding of both the individual and the therapist. Together, each is healed in the therapeutic experience. Having been dean of a medical school, a practicing and teaching psychiatrist, and an ordained Methodist minister, Dr. James Knight is in the unique position of reflecting the physical, mental, and spiritual dimensions in his training and work, sharing with us his view of the opportunity open to us to direct our lives into channels that can bring us greater meaning.

It is rare, but fortunately less so as time goes on, to encounter a man who is the dean of a medical school, trained in the rigors of scientific medicine, who appreciates aspects of the art of medical care and is in a position to help balance a medical education program to accommodate a greater breadth of thought. Dr. Robert Liebelt is an unusual man, and he brings great vision to his ideas about the global approach to health and about his school's contribution in training the physician of tomorrow—today.

We wonder who to consult and where to go for help when we become ill. With such a multitude of services and qualified personnel to be able to consult, how does one decide who to see—physician, specialist, hospital, clergyman, psychotherapist, and on and on? Dr. Donald Hayes, a sensitive humanistic physician who appreciates the dilemma, makes some helpful suggestions about where to go and who to see to help yourself if you become ill.

Believing that "lessons learned from the dying can and do provide the courage for the living to face their inner fears . . . the 'little' deaths of life's transitions," Dr. Elisabeth Kübler-Ross shares some of her insights in the Epilogue. Her scientific and humanitarian work in the field of death and dying has opened up new opportunities for a greater understanding of human existence and has caused many people to reconsider their thoughts about the meaning of death—viewing it not as the end but rather as part of the process of transition.

The first as well as the final chapter outlines my own experiences and my perspective about where we are now, about what the future can be like, and about the exciting prospects for change—change that each of us can and must make if we are to grow and enrich our lives. I assume full responsibility for these chapters and would not want to convey the impression that they are necessarily the views of any of my associate contributors.

I was trained as a psychologist and have been a business

executive for some years. The past nine years have given me an opportunity to learn, to grow, and to share the experiences of several thousand people who came to a holistic health center, Renaissance, Revitalization Center in Nassau, Bahamas. Having Having cofounded this center with my brother, a physician who contributor to this book, and my associate and good friend, a European physician, Dr. Ivan Popov, I have had the chance to see how many possible ways there are to help people help themselves. I have learned what humanity in medicine is all about from the application of the rich and varied experiences of Dr. Popov; how traditional and responsible nontraditional methods could work together to create a healing environment in which people could help re-establish harmony and balance in their lives; and how I, in counseling with clients, could share what I knew from my own personal experiences and training.

My aim in this book has been to call upon the range of that training and experience to synthesize the three descriptive aspects of man—body, mind, and spirit—specifically related to his health and disease. Some of my own theoretical notions have been advanced. I am most conscious of the deficiencies of such a position, since it is not easy to document the data on which some of my thinking is based.

Bringing this fine array of loving, caring people together has been a rewarding and happy experience for me. It has enriched my life to know them all, and my sincere and deep appreciation is extended to them for taking time out of their busy schedules to participate in this book.

I invite you now to share with me the many inspiring thoughts you will find within—so that we may both experience being healed together.

Acknowledgments

So many people have touched my life to bring this book into being, it is not possible to list them all. Some have had a direct involvement with this project, however, and I would like to express my appreciation to them.

Thanks to my friend Richard Weiner who first suggested the idea of my doing a book and encouraged me to do it. Thanks also to Michael Hunter, my editor at Prentice-Hall, for his early confidence and interest in publishing it.

I am deeply grateful to the many people in Houston, Texas, who offered me their friendship and love in support of my efforts there during the past four years. It has been a truly remarkable experience for me to see the holistic health activity grow from an idea to an active organization providing meaningful educational activities for people in Texas. The Holistic Health Association has enabled me to meet and know many find people—among them some of the contributors of this book.

My sincere thanks to Dorothy Goldenfarb, Sheila Schneider, and Sandra Knowles for helping type parts of the manuscript and to Virginia Fife for her help and radiant smiles of encouragement. To Virginia Jewett, always available for last-minute typing to meet deadlines, goes my sincerest thanks. Appreciation to my friend Harold Kintz for many fruitful hours of conversation that provided valuable insights. My appreciation to Dr. Grant Taylor, whose wisdom and humanity provided me with many suggestions and ideas. I truly value his advice and friendship. Without the interest, generosity, and friendship of Robert Gantt many of my undertakings in Houston would not have been realized, including this book. My dear friend, Holly Cravens, assisted in so many ways. She is a truly beautiful person who gave me continuous encouragement and editorial help at important moments. Thanks to Ovid DaSilva for his contribution.

To my friends and associates of Renaissance, Dr. Ivan Popov and Dr. Fred Hering, goes my appreciation for valuable suggestions that help improve the manuscript. I am grateful to the many clients of Renaissance who over the past eight years have shared so many of their experiences with me. I learned many important lessons during the sessions we spent together.

To my children, Alison and Jon. Their love and belief in their father have been a constant source of strength for me. Special thanks to Jon for enduring the reading of proofs with me.

My eternal gratitude to Helen, Bill, Jerry, Judy, Bob, and Ken, with whom I have shared *A Course in Miracles,* an extraordinary experience that has helped me understand the meaning of my life.

Without the dedicated collaboration of the contributors to this book, my ambitions for it would not have been realized. I thank them sincerely for joining me in this enriching experience. In particular, I wish to thank Dr. Hans Selye for his appreciation of the book's concept and his remarkable insights that continue to reaffirm the significance of his life's work on stress as the basis of disease and illness. I predict that his contributions will affect the focus of medicine and health care for generations to come. The time we shared together was most rewarding and gave me an appreciation of his eminent capacity to achieve a balance of the specialist and generalist.

I reserve a special expression of appreciation for Wil Lepkowski, senior editor of *Chemical and Engineering News,* whose awareness and professional competence were so valuable in the editorial assistance he gave me. He raised pertinent questions, caused me to refine my thinking, and challenged me to distill the essence of my ideas. I appreciate our friendship, and the periodic dialogues we have shared have been a most gratifying experience for me.

Contributors

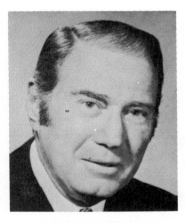

MALCOLM TODD, M.D., Past president of the American Medical Association (1974–1975) and California Medical Association, is Clinical Professor of Surgery, University of California (Irvine) and Fellow, American College of Surgeons, past President International College of Surgeons and American College of Gastroenterology. He was a United States delegate to the World Health Organization, Geneva, Switzerland 1970, 1971, and 1972.

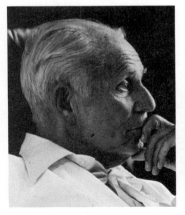

HANS SELYE, Ph.D., M.D., D.Sc., is Emeritus Professor at the University of Montreal and President of the International Institute of Stress. He has written over 38 books, including the classic, *The Stress of Life*. He holds earned and honorary doctorates in medicine, philosophy, and science. He is a Fellow of the Royal Society of Canada and has been made a Companion of the Order of Canada, the highest decoration awarded by his country.

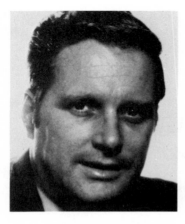

CHARLES F. STROEBEL, Ph.D., M.D., is Associate Director of Research and Director of Psychophysiology Laboratories and Clinic at the Institute of Living, Hartford. He is on the faculty of the Department of Psychiatry, Yale University Medical School, Professor of Psychiatry at the University of Connecticut Health Center and Medical School, and Professor of Bioengineering at Trinity College.

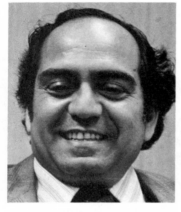

SYED ABDULLAH, M.D., is a diplomate of the American Board of Psychiatry and Neurology, and staff psychiatrist at Rockland Psychiatric Center, Orangeburg, N.Y. He also teaches clinical psychiatry at Columbia University, and he has a private practice in New York City.

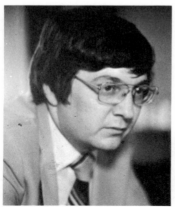

O. CARL SIMONTON, M.D., D.A.B.R., Director, Cancer Counseling and Research Center, Forth Worth, Texas. Dr. Simonton and Stephanie Matthews–Simonton have developed a new approach to cancer treatment combining traditional treatment methods with meditation techniques and psychotherapy.

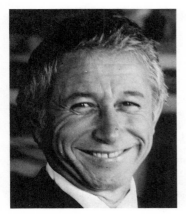

GERALD G. JAMPOLSKY, M.D. Dr. Jampolsky is a psychiatrist, formerly on the faculty of University of California Medical Center, San Francisco, founder of and now consultant to The Center for Attitudinal Healing in Tiburon, California. He has been engaged in working with children who have cancer and is achieving remarkable results with alternative healing methods.

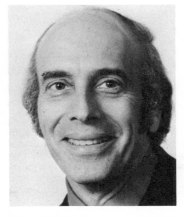

WILLIAM J. GOLDWAG, M.D., is now in the private practice of preventive medicine in southern California. Formerly faculty member of Long Island University, he writes a column on nutrition for *Bestways* magazine and a syndicated newspaper column.

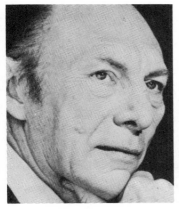

MARCUS BACH, Ph.D., is the author of 20 books and founder and director of the Fellowship for Spiritual Understanding in Palos Verdes Estates, California. Dr. Bach is a most sought-after speaker in the field of human potential and total health. He was formerly Professor of Comparative Religion at the University of Iowa and holds four honorary degrees from other universities.

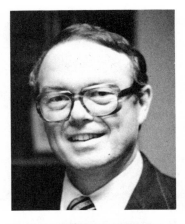

JULIAN BYRD, S.T.M. Director of Pastoral Care and Education at Hermann Hospital, Houston, Texas, has spent many years in personal pastoral counseling in hospital settings. He was formerly Director of the Institute of Religion and Chief Chaplain at M.D. Anderson Hospital, University of Texas Medical Center, Houston.

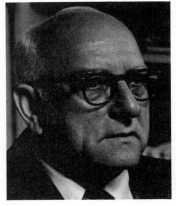

JAMES A. KNIGHT, M.D., is Professor of Psychiatry, Louisiana State University School of Medicine and formerly Professor of Psychiatry and Dean of Texas A&M College of Medicine. Author of eight books and numerous articles in varied publications, Dr. Knight is also an ordained Methodist minister.

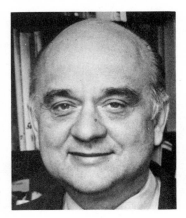

ROBERT L. LIEBELT, Ph.D., M.D. is Dean of the Northeastern Ohio Universities College of Medicine. Dr. Liebelt has an outstanding career as a medical educator with several medical schools and has served on numerous public commissions in medicine. He has written more than 100 scientific papers and is one of the leaders in helping to improve medical education in the United States.

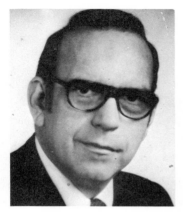

DONALD M. HAYES, M.D., is Professor and Chairman, Department of Community Medicine, University of Texas Medical School, Houston, Texas. Dr. Hayes is a Consultant to the National Science Foundation and the National Cancer Institute and was formerly Associate Dean for Community Health Sciences of Bowman Gray School of Medicine. He has written numerous scientific papers and a book entitled *Between Doctor and Patient.*

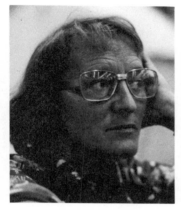

ELISABETH KÜBLER-ROSS, M.D., is Founder and Chairman of the Board of Shanti Nilaya, a growth center in Escondido, California. She was formerly Assistant Professor of Psychiatry at the University of Chicago Medical School and is internationally known for her scientific and humanitarian work in the field of death and dying. Dr. Ross holds 13 honorary doctorate degrees, as well as numerous other awards and honors. She is the author of four books, among them the well-known *Death, The Final Stage of Growth** and her latest, *To Live Until We Say Good-Bye*

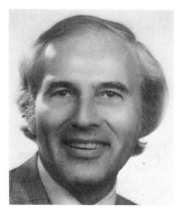

ELLIOTT M. GOLDWAG is the co-founder of the Renaissance Revitalization Center, Nassau, Bahamas. He is the founder and Executive Director of Holistic Health Association, Houston, Texas, and he has written numerous articles on health subjects.

*Also published by Prentice-Hall, Inc.

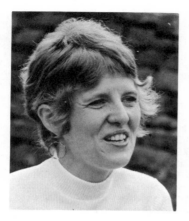

VALORY MURRAY is coordinator of a teaching and research program in geriatric medicine and gerontology being developed at Northeastern Ohio Universities College of Medicine. She is a Ph.D. candidate at Kent State University.

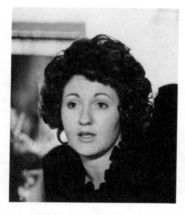

STEPHANIE MATTHEWS-SIMONTON is a founder and Director of Counseling at the Cancer Counseling and Research Center in Fort Worth, Texas. She has developed and implemented a psychotherapy training program for cancer counselors and is co-author of the book, *Getting Well Again.*

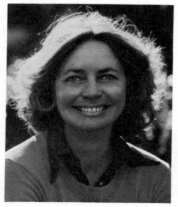

PATRICIA TAYLOR is a founder and coordinator of children's programs at the Center For Attitudinal Healing in Tiburon, California. She established a pen pal/phone pal network putting children with catastrophic illness, in touch with each other around the country.

Introduction

The Challenge to Medicine: Prevention of Illness

MALCOLM TODD, M.D.

Some of my colleagues in organized medicine may think it strange that one of its leaders—through my introduction to this book—has become identified with the subject of total, or holistic health—the integration of body, mind, and spirit. But to me, it seems very proper and timely that the medical profession, its related organizations, and the public at large should become informed and involved in new alternative programs of health care.

It is for these reasons that I am so honored and willing to be associated with this book and with its authors. Their work, described in these pages, points the way to establishing strong clinical bases to those alternative therapies. New knowledge of the health care process can only help organized medicine and conventional practitioners do their own curative jobs better and with less stress.

Physicians already admit there should be alternatives to the traditional management of disease, of life, and of death and dying. We know there is need for lifestyle modification in dealing with stress and tension. Research could show that there may actually be a new perspective on the treatment of organic illness, but these modalities of treatment must have a scientific basis. We need to learn and evaluate lifetime modification skills derived from ancient cultural traditions. The difficulty, but the necessity, is to learn to integrate them with today's new technological discoveries.

The responsibilities of a physician to his patient were clearly outlined by Hippocrates more than 2,300 years ago when he emphasized that the physician must consider the *whole* man in order to diagnose and treat health care problems properly. He pointed out that the well-being of man is influenced by social and environmental, as well as physiological changes, and that the art and science of medicine includes considerations of all these factors.

The original Hippocratic Oath bids the physician to swear by "Appollo the physician, and Aesculapius and Hygeia and Panacea. . . . " Hygeia, of course, is synonymous with the prevention of disease and calls on the physician to be concerned with preventive as well as therapeutic medicine. Preventive medicine was reinforced in the Hippocratic Doctrines, which stated that "The well-being of man is influenced by all environmental factors . . . that quality of air, water, and food, the winds and topography of the land . . . and the general living habits."

But Hippocrates lived in much simpler times—long before the revolution in medical science and technology brought forth the allopathic approach to medicine with its emphasis on treatment of disease rather than the more Hippocratic approach of prevention. This revolution has allowed medicine to address itself to the mechanistic processes of disease and death with a dazzling genius unparalleled in the history of mankind.

Through advances in vaccines and antibiotics, it has eliminated many serious diseases and moderated scores of others. It has developed undreamed of surgical and clinical capabilities and has created the finest quality medical care system in the world.

But this revolution has also brought problems as well as progress. In our preoccupation with the quality of care, we have failed to pay proper attention to the *costs* and the *accessibility* of care. In our emphasis on the therapeutic aspects of care, we have neglected the individual social and environmental stress factors in disease causation. And finally, because of the much heavier demands placed on his time and energy by modern medicine and by rising public expectations, the individual physician finds it difficult to make a significant contribution to the larger profession. The World Health Organization's preamble defines health as "a state of complete physical, mental, and social well-being and not merely the absence of disease or infirmity." So it should be to this end that we work as we try to improve the quality of life of all our people.

There can be no doubt that our society has passed through the golden age of medicine. This period began in the mid 1930s with specialization in medical care. Blood banks and transfusions, antibiotics, anesthesiology, improved nursing care, open heart surgery, organ transplants, and radioisotopes: All have played a vital role. Perhaps our next age will reward us with the long-awaited victory over cancer, an understanding of genetic diseases, the chemical treatment of mental illness, a mechanical heart and other devices, immunotherapy to combat infections, and the like. But as we aspire to achieve these accomplishments, we should consider the question of whether our enchantment over dramatic and rare surgery or our need to compete for the bigger and better breakthrough in "conquering" a disease made us less eager to work on prevention.

We might ask ourselves whether our success in kidney transplants for chronic kidney disease justified the risk and complications of the technical procedure and thus whether, instead, we should be concentrating on the early detection and management of urinary tract infections. We might also ask whether we should continue coronary bypass operations, or whether, instead, we should develop better detection and medical treatment of patients with coronary insufficiency. Perhaps our efforts should be designed toward finding the causes of degenerative diseases rather than perfecting total hip and joint replacements and knee prostheses.

What I am saying, obviously, is that we begin pursuing with intelligence and good will some of the more promising avenues in holistic care. Along with waging that war on cancer . . . or on heart disease . . . or on arthritis, should we not also mount an assault on stress? Up to now, stress has been regarded almost perfunctorily among the body of practitioners, perhaps because it has been so much a part of their own daily work experience.

I believe everyone should be interested in the emerging concept of holistic health and what it entails. We might begin by asking:

What is holistic health?

What is scientifically involved in the holistic view of medicine?

Is it just a curious and exotic term, or are there real values in this approach to health?

Is there now a need for holistic health in our society?

Enthusiasm for quick and easy solutions to serious, long-term problems is one of the lesser qualities of civilization. Thus, although many aspects of holistic health excite me, especially those that promise to introduce concepts and practices that could creatively revise current patterns of disease causation, I bring caution to it as well. I need to know whether all the elements of antistress practices are scientifically sound. And I am concerned that they fit into our traditional pattern of health care. For it is in no one's interest to upset or to undermine a specialized medicine that has proven its own scientific success in understanding and relieving disorder after disorder.

With that caveat, I can turn to holistic health with considerable enthusiasm and expectation.

Dr. Richard Svihus, speaking on the origin and definition of holistic health, recalls that the first reference in the literature to its meaning is found in the 1974 edition of the *Encyclopedia Britannica*. It defined holism as: "The philosophical theory, based on the presupposition of emergent evaluation, that entirely new things or wholes are produced by a creative form within the universe. They are consequently more than mere rearrangements of particles that already exist. In other words, an entity is greater in its wholeness than the sum of its parts, and a new plateau of existence is reached when this new wholeness is obtained."

R. A. Chilgren, M.D., an associate professor of pediatrics at the University of Minnesota, has written me:

> The term "holistic health" in some ways is really a catchall for alternative approaches to health. But there is an implied, if not specific, direction. This direction, already moving in many places, might be reflected by the term "integration of mind, body, and spirit," or by redefining health in the sense of including consciousness raising or growth. . . .
>
> On the other hand, in a more ethical sense it addresses the human energy crisis, the energy-sapping lifestyle problems or critical life events less amenable to a technologic approach to medicine. It redirects us to the importance of exploring our inner space or consciousness, as well as outer space, through emphasis on health education and responsibility for self.

We physicians need to reassess the total health of our individual patients and, in turn, that of our entire society. In this way, *all* people may benefit from the cultural and environmental as well as the physical and mental advances. Further, it seems not unreasonable that physicians must engage sooner or later in practice patterns that integrate physical, mental, spiritual, and environmental health in some comprehensive manner. This is what I think holistic health means. The entire system from the politics to the practice of medicine will benefit.

Since the late 1950s and 1960s, a goal of the American Medical Association has been to develop a program integrating the body, mind, and spirit in the treatment of the whole patient. This was a part of our program of medicine and religion, and considerable progress has ensued. In the process, it has been suggested that all modalities of treatment may be used in holistic healing—surgery, medicine, chemotherapy, radiation, nutrition, rehabilitation, and—yes—hypnosis, acupuncture, parapsychology, and, of course, religion.

In order to achieve such a broad goal, it will be necessary to tap the resources of our most learned scholars, our most sophisticated researchers, and our expert clinicians and practitioners. For that ultimate goal is to use these authorities to teach an individual to assume responsibility for himself and to heal himself through the modification of any unhealthy attitudes, values, or lifestyles.

So far, I believe it is apparent that the spectrum of components of holistic health is as wide as the number of people you may ask. The range might be from biofeedback, biorhythm, and psychology of consciousness to paranormal phenomena and psychic healing. There is also obviously a wide range of competency—from the solid, scientific, and reliable to downright fakery and quackery. We find it in holistic medicine, but we find it, too, in conventional medicine. My point is that there is no substitute for effective thought and professional integrity.

Menninger implies in his writings that the inability of doctors and psychiatrists to practice medicine that integrates the body, mind, and the environment is striking. Resistance on the part of the medical profession to these new approaches may be due to one or two conceptual polarities in medicine—that is, body-mind dualism, and the separation of health from illness.

If this is holistic medicine, and if it does merit a place in our society, then doctors should take the lead to see that the expansion and growth of the concept takes place in a responsible manner. Of course, it will not replace traditional medicine, but it might very well complement and become an integral part of traditional practice.

There are many factors outside the province of medicine that play significant roles in undermining our quality of life—poverty, unemployment, malnutrition and subnutrition, morality, crime, divorce, human unhappiness, and stress. Especially stress, for that causes a multitude of pathological conditions.

We have all learned that certain stress factors in our lives contribute to many physical problems. It is agreed that the more we know about ourselves—our body, our psyche, our illness, and our environment—the better prepared we are to take personal responsibility for our health by understanding stress, reducing it, and obtaining optimum health.

Disciplining our own lives against the abuse of our bodies and minds, evaluating our moral and ethical standards of living, and, ultimately, eliminating poverty will do much to improve our quality of life.

In recent years, more and more attention has been focused on health education. This is. as it should be. There has been, of course, a renewed interest in preventive care. This interest goes far beyond the scope of the traditional immunizations and innoculations that form the basis for any preventive care program.

During the past ten years, much has been written and spoken about preventive care. As a matter of fact, the provision of preventive care is one of the requirements by law of all health maintenance organizations. Yet none of them, to my knowledge, really offers true preventive services. Yes, they provide shots and immunizations, and some have multiphasic screening programs; but real preventive medicine involves the individual as well as the provider, and it begins with health education.

Since the turn of the century, present health education needs have emerged from four major developments.

1. The emergence of major disease problems intimately related to patterns of living learned early in life.
2. Emergence of a health care delivery system that depends for its successful functioning on informed and motivated consumers.
3. The emergence of the idea that health is a state of total positive functioning in informed and motivated consumers.
4. The emergence of an ecological view of the world that sees man synergistically and simultaneously related to all of his environment.

In the early part of this century, the major threats to life and health were communicable diseases caused by specific pathogens. Today, the communicable diseases are largely under control, and chronic degenerative diseases and accidents have become the major health problems. These are conditions that have no single cause but stem in large part from learned patterns of living adhered to over periods of many years. The next twenty years will be a transition period as the focus of health care moves from crisis intervention and the cure of disease to the maintenance of optimum physical and mental health and disease prevention.

It is very obvious that there is a need for coordinated comprehensive health education programs in schools, colleges, and communities, as well as in health care delivery systems. Dangerous and apparently illogical health behavior appears as such only from the detached, rational, scientific view the health professional assumes when he judges the health behavior of others. Such behavior may appear logical and necessary when viewed from inside the consumer's—and, indeed, the health professional's—own inner world of needs. We must break that cycle of thought where "need" amounts to self-destructive behavior through mounting stress patterns.

In 1978, Americans spent $10 billion on tobacco and $10.5 billion on alcohol. Thirty-five million people will be taking stimulants and tranquilizers. Forty million Americans will spend over one billion dollars trying to control their weight. In other words, a big percentage of the nation's sickness and death is a fault, at least in part, of the patients themselves. And, yes, 60,000 Americans will die in automobile accidents in 1979, and probably half of those accidents will be due to alcohol. We are living in a "modern" society in which affluence, convenience, and stress conspire to place us where we become increasing risks to chronic and degenerative diseases.

It has been said that the goal of holistic health is a promotion of vigorous well-being. Perhaps one might say that holistic health is an individual commitment. Actually, it seems to me that this concept could well supplement our many problem areas in therapy. But it is up to each of us as individuals to make the changes in our lifestyles and in our environment that bring about good health. Many people suffering from functional illnesses or from those symptoms that accompany organic diseases insist that they want to get well but unconsciously enjoy byproducts of an illness such as sympathy, special attention, shared responsibility, and punishment from guilt. Some psychologists say there is a limit to the benefits received from medical care if you don't respect the possibility of unconscious processes playing a role in your illnesses.

Acupuncture, biofeedback, hypnotism, homeopathy, herbalism, and meditation have indeed found a place in holistic medicine. Now we need to begin ferreting out the effective from the fraudulent—just as we must continuously do in the medicine we already know. For a person in either psychic or physical pain is calling for help and, too often, is susceptible to offers of a quick or magical cure. The source for cure, we now know, is the self. Ideally, the physician and healer is a teacher who brings the patient to a realization of his strength and wholeness.

Several years ago, it was my privilege to head the American Medical Association delegation to visit the People's Republic of China. There, we saw the many benefits of public health in a controlled, regulated, and disciplined society. We, of course, studied acupuncture, moxibustion, and pharmacological potions. We also saw, firsthand, the Chinese emphasis on preventive care. And we were reminded of an old Chinese adage: "The superior physician treats the patient before the illness is manifested. It is only the inferior physician who treats the illness he was unable to prevent." This, of course, could be interpreted as the first form of holistic medicine.

In the future, the well-being of mankind will depend to a large extent on the successful education of consumers and professionals alike. Perhaps there is now a need for a truly comprehensive system—a new conceptual model of understanding, diagnosis, prevention, and treatment of illness—to be achieved through education. I consider this book to be a strong start toward that new basis.

1

The Dilemma
In Health Care

ELLIOTT M. GOLDWAG, PH.D.

According to the latest United States government health statistics, the daily cost of a hospital stay is now more than $200 versus $40 in 1965. In 1950, the total cost of medical care in the Unites States was $12 billion. Now it is more than $200 billion.

About twenty million Americans take barbiturates, thirty million are on tranquilizers, and 600 tons of sleeping pills are consumed each year, or roughly thirty million doses each night.

A Public Health Service study in 1976 estimated that 25.2 million people, or 12.7 percent of the population, had some limitation in their activities due to a chronic disease condition. Forty million persons have some form of heart and blood vessel disease, three million suffer from cancer, 31 million endure the pain of arthritis and rheumatism, 21 million carry an ulcer.

To "endure" and to "suffer"—that seems to be the pattern of thought in a society that expects and accepts illness much as it does the rising and setting of the sun.

Defenders of the current health system point to an eighteen-year gain in life expectancy at birth since 1900. But we shouldn't be fooled by that statistic. The average American's life expectancy past the age of forty-five, according to Dr. Rene Dubos of Rockefeller University, "is hardly greater today than it was several decades ago and is shorter than that of many European people of the present generation."

Dr. Dubos says that the average American may claim the highest standard of living in the world. But ten percent of his income already goes for medical care. That same American, says Dr. Dubos (1959), "cannot build hospitals fast enough to accommodate the sick. He is encouraged to believe that money can create drugs for the cure of heart disease, cancer, and mental disease. But he makes no worthwhile effort to recognize, let alone correct, the mismanagements of his everyday life that contribute to the high incidence of these conditions."

Dr. Richard E. Palmer, past president of the American Medical Association, cites an article stating that more medical care does not equal health: "The best estimates are that the medical system . . . affects about 10% of the usual indices for measuring health . . . .The remaining 90% are determined by factors over which doctors have little or no control."

We have become overwhelmed, many feel, with the scientific technology of medicine and have forgotten the patient in the process. He has been reduced, as Dr. Liebelt reminds us, to "chronic livers" or "bad hearts" or to a group of parts and pieces that has come in for a repair job on one of its faulty mechanisms.

Dr. Robert Moser (1976), former editor of the official *Journal of the American Medical Association*, offers a further evaluation of the current system.

I think we are better listeners to organs (especially hearts) than the good clinicians of earlier days. However, they were better listeners to patients. I suspect some atrophy of our diagnostic senses occurred when subjective observation . . . was replaced by objective laboratory data.

It would appear that we need to be reminded of some things history teaches us but which we seem to have forgotten in these past 100 years of "advanced" medical technology and sophistication. The basic principles go back to Hippocrates, the father of modern medicine, after whom every physician swears an oath when he obtains his medical degree. Hippocrates was an exponent of the idea that the natural healing force within each person is the greatest factor in getting well. He said it was the physician's duty to work with Nature and to enhance those healing forces so that they could work in harmonious fashion. Using as healing media the natural elements of sea water, fresh air, exercise, and diet, Hippocrates' emphasis was on the person, not the condition.

Health achieved as a balance of processes was an idea of the ancients from Galen right into more modern times. The Greeks identified it as "physis," meaning the bond between man and environment. Constant challenges from the environment have disturbed the balance and provoked ill health and disease. The organism had the ability to deal with those disturbances and recover naturally. This was the *vis medicatrix natural* of Hippocrates. Today, it is called adapting and coping.

Today, we seem to deify disease and illness with grand edifices called hospitals and medical centers, with large amounts of dollars for developing new technologies to probe our ailing organs, and with drugs to chase away viruses, germs, bacteria, and other noxious agents. We have let ourselves be mesmerized into thinking we have a health care system, when actually what we really have is a disease care model.

We have been led to believe that we can buy relief and prevention at a doctor's office and at the pharmacy. We believe that research is the answer to conquering diseases, but we have failed to accept or recognize the most important factor in health care: that it is up to the individual to take responsibility for his own health. We seem to be on that never-ending search for the molecular cause of every illness, and we seem to think that as soon as that cause is discovered, all the problems of illness will be solved. We have come to place our faith and trust in what scientists and medical professionals believe to be true, attributing to them the infallible opinion that if they believe it to be true, it must be true, or otherwise they would not hold to that opinion.

We consumers of health find it easy to blame physicians for their lack of caring and for their dehumanized attitudes in the way they practice their science. But at the same time, we are being poor physicians to ourselves when we continue to lead a debilitating lifestyle; when we harbor anger, fear, and resentments in our daily life; when we drive eighty miles an hour, stuff ourselves with worthless junk food, drink ourselves into a stupor, or smoke like a human chimney.

The Canadian government has devoted a great deal of time and attention to developing an improved system of health care. Dr. Thomas Boudreau (1975), Assistant Deputy Minister of Health, has stated that the health status of each person is related to three main elements: (1) lifestyle; (2) environment, both physical and social; and (3) human biology. He points out that the five main causes of early death, calculated against life expectancy, are:

1. Car accidents—12%
2. Disease—11%
3. Other accidents—10%
4. Respiratory problems and cancer—8%
5. Suicide—4.1%

Biomedical research will not provide the main answers to these problems. These are problems that reflect lifestyle. But for us to take responsibility for maintaining our health involves profound changes in our way of perceiving the world and our own attitudes toward it. Most of us have grown up abdicating our responsibility and have passed it over to the doctor, to Medicare, to Blue Cross, or to whatever else is around to take care of us and to help foot the bill. Thus we have erroneously placed our dependence on the system and its chief representative, the physician. When we begin hurting again, we return to the chief magician, the doctor, who has an exotic array of needles, pills, potions, and knives for repairing our damaged parts in order to make everything go away. The result is the creation of a dependency relationship rather than a creative, cooperative effort between physician and patient.

Dependency can extend beyond the physician to include medications. For example, one of the great contributions of medical science has been the discovery of insulin for diabetes. Prior to this, diabetics would frequently go into coma and die. Insulin has permitted people to live out lives they would never have enjoyed. However, a common belief is that the cause of diabetes is improper secretion of insulin from the pancreas. Right? Wrong! The inability of the pancreas to secrete proper amounts of insulin is a description of a process or mechanism. Dubos (1959) very pointedly discusses this subject:

> . . . The story of insulin and diabetes well illustrates that the discovery of a therapeutic agent does not necessarily solve the problem of disease causation. . . . The primary disturbance may be in some part of the body quite remote from the pancreas and the deficiency of insulin may be secondary to it . . . . Unfortunately, effective control of the symptoms of diabetes is not synonymous with cure of the diabetic patient, let alone with conquest of the disease.

One might be led to the conclusion that I am opposed to the use of drugs. On the contrary, sulfa drugs, for example, have proved to be a major relief in many illnesses for which we are inadequately prepared. And anti-biotics have saved many lives which otherwise could have been lost. One simply needs to put the use of drugs in proper perspective. They should be considered as *temporary* solutions to acute medical intervention; they should be used for the removal of symptoms, not for dealing with the more basic causes that lie within our belief systems. If drugs were the cure, the same drug would work for everyone in a given condition. Every physician knows this is not so. It is also true that when parts have degenerated beyond repair or when accidents create trauma that needs mending, surgery is a necessary and welcome mode of treatment. But what do we do to keep that person from getting into another crisis? And what do we do to prevent people from reaching the point of crisis in the first place? Let's briefly examine what I believe are the antecedents to the current health care system.

In the nineteenth century, the work of Louis Pasteur produced what we know today as the "germ theory of disease." This theory proposed that illness or disease is caused by one or more germs, viruses, or bacteria that invade the organism and wreak their havoc upon the unprotected victim. This belief became very popular among medical and scientific thought of the day. It was a clearly articulated position that problems of illness and disease are outside the skin. Thus, the familiar phrases of "doing battle with the enemy," "war on disease," and "invasion of bacteria" became battle cries reminiscent of strife between opposing forces.

The natural consequence of the germ theory is that if germs cause disease, then they must be destroyed. Therefore, it would be logical to find "destroyer" agents that would knock out the enemy before it had a chance to devour us. Accordingly, the emphasis began to focus on finding drugs to kill these rascals. And we really did go at it with a great deal of fervor and enthusiasm, until today we are able to boast of perhaps 200,000 or more drugs and chemicals to kill the "invaders" or disrupters of our peace of body and mind.

A contemporary of Pasteur was an equally famous French scientist by the name of Claude Bernard. Bernard (1927) had a different view of the same problem. Being a physiologist (unlike Pasteur, who was a bacteriologist), he proposed that the "germ," "virus," or "bacteria" was not the problem but rather the "interior milieu" or internal environment in which the germs found themselves. If the internal conditions were fertile enough for germs to flourish and do their damage, then disease would be the result. If, however, the internal environment of our body was in proper balance, functioning in equilibrium, then such germs could not find a "happy hunting ground" and would be eliminated by the system or remain innocuous.

Needless to say, the germ theory was the position adopted by most people, and modern medicine took off from there. Pasteur is purported to have said on his deathbed, however: "Bernard was right. It is not the germ but the internal milieu."

Even Rudolf Virchow (1958), the father of scientific medicine, upon which our current medical thinking is based, discarded the idea that the germ is primary.

> As soon as one is convinced that there are no disease entities one must realize that no therapeutic entities can be set up in opposition to them . . . . If disease is only the orderly manifestation of definite phenomena of life (normal in themselves) under unusual conditions, with deviations which are simply quantitative, then all therapy must be essentially directed against the altered conditions . . . .

And recently, Dr. Lewis Thomas (1974), head of the prestigious Sloan-Kettering Cancer Memorial Hospital, also questioned our focus on germs. In discussing the numerous kinds of bacteria and germs that inhabit the surface as well as internal parts of the human body, he describes their role this way:

> The micro-organisms that seem to have it in for us in the worst way—the ones that really appear to wish us ill—turn out on close examination to be rather more like bystanders, strays, strangers in from the cold. They will invade and replicate if given the chance, and some of them will get into our deepest tissues and set forth in the blood, but it is our response to their presence that makes the disease. Our arsenals for fighting off bacteria are so powerful, and involve so many different defense mechanisms, that we are in more danger from them than from the invaders.

The experience many researchers and physicians have had with the so-called "placebo" effect is probably the most single important contradiction of the germ theory of disease. The administration of ordinary sugar pills in place of some real medication (without the patient's knowledge) continues to produce a remarkable relief of symptoms in a significant number of patients.

In one reported study in 1956, it was found that of 1,000 patients treated, 35.2% obtained satisfactory relief from the symptoms studied by being given an innocuous pill. The symptoms included severe postoperative wound pain, the pain of angina pectoris, headache, cough, mood change, seasickness, anxiety, and the common cold (Beecher, 1956). In another more recent study, Haas, Fink, and Hartfelder (1963) reported that out of 14,177 patients with various ills, 40.6% obtained relief from the placebo (sugar pills). This means that patients who *thought* they were given medication for their problem actually received a sugar pill.

I believe this is one of the best demonstrations that the "placebo" effect is more of what Dr. Jerome Frank (1973) has called the "faith" effect—the belief system of these patients in the physician or his agent that the drug being given would help them feel better. I believe, furthermore, that if the strength of a person's belief in the doctor and what he suggests will relieve the illness is stronger than the pathogen which provoked the illness, the patient will obtain relief from his symptoms, and the relief will last as long as the strength of the belief is maintained.

The germ theory has a number of other counterparts that relate to this system of thought about science and the world. Inherited from that same late nineteenth century era is a particular view of the human organism and how it functions, known as the "reductionist" approach—sometimes referred to as "elementalist," "analytical," or "inductive." This means that in trying to understand how a thing works, you take it apart to get a better knowledge of how the pieces work. Then you divide these pieces into small subpieces and continue to look at these fragments. After a while, you become so infatuated with the pieces and subpieces that you may have forgotten the purpose for which you began the study in the first place. Also, the logic of the detailed working parts seems like the reason the whole thing works; that is, until you find another part and go further. This is what may be happening with many of our scientific explorations. They encourage a tendency to look at piecemeal units, at isolated variables, sometimes measuring a single variable at a time.

What we are saying is that this approach tends to view the body as a machine engineered to a certain precision; when it is out of order, it is taken to a specialist to fix the part. All persons who fit the description of the machine are treated with the same standard accepted method. Since something "out there" is making your organ ill, something "out there" in the form of treatment will make you well—something prescribed by someone "out there."

This fragmentation of man has led to a separation consciousness. It has further encouraged alienation in our society, generating fear and loneliness. Such preoccupation has removed the soul of man and separated him from his God by seeing him as pieces and parts different from one another.

The alternative to this analytic approach is known as "integrative," "holistic," "synthetic," or "deductive." Here, the aim is to understand the living organism as a total entity and to understand its parts as integrated, interdependent, interrelated systems that can be understood by studying the parts, but without losing sight of their relation to the whole organism.

Thus, we can describe a human being in a variety of ways in terms of subjective experience, physiological function, biochemical composition, or anatomic structure. No description is any more "fundamental" than any other. Each is a focus on the whole man.

Bernard's theory of the internal environment follows this holistic model more closely. It also parallels the thought of the ancients who recognized man's relationship with the cosmos and the natural order of all life. In their ideal, they adhered to the practice of certain natural laws that maintained harmony and ecological balance in the Universe. Certainly, Bernard's contribution becomes more significant as we reassert the balance between science and art, recognizing that they are not adversaries but part of the same spectrum of human creativity.

Bernard's twentieth-century counterpart was Walter B. Cannon, a well-known physiologist and physician who taught at Harvard Medical School for many years. It was Cannon who developed the now universally accepted concept of "homeostasis" in his well-known book, *The Wisdom of the Body* (1939).

Cannon postulated in 1926 that the body, being composed of unstable material and subjected to continuous disturbing conditions, has internal regulators that are always acting to maintain a constant state of equilibrium. Any tendency toward change is automatically met with increasing strength from the factors that resist change. When a factor is known which can shift the homeostatic state in one direction, we can look for factors that have the opposite effect. We have regulators that maintain the internal environment, so that fluctuations occur within narrow limits in response to internal or external disturbances. Many simultaneous processes occur, each affecting the other and providing a continuous feedback in order to maintain balance.

There have been studies to demonstrate this regulatory process—the body's consciousness of health. For example, in some individuals, exercise increases thyroid function, while in others it has the opposite effect. The object, obviously, is not to reduce or increase any function other than what the body knows to be normal for that person. Both Bernard and Cannon recognized the importance of all forces in the body working in an intimate relationship to keep all functioning within very narrow limits of disruption in order to maintain equilibrium and a positive internal environment. They saw the biological function as an integrated whole, each part dependent upon the other for its synchronicity, requiring no conscious effort on our part to maintain coordination and automatic functioning.

While Claude Bernard was making his important theory public, Sigmund Freud (1943), originally a neurophysiologist, was introducing his theory of the unconscious influences responsible for behavior and for certain types of illness. His work produced that monumental contribution to the medical and lay world called psychoanalysis. Like Bernard's, Freud's system postulated an internal set of forces of the mind (as distinct from the body organ known as the brain) called id, ego, and superego—forces that formed the early years of childhood and programmed patterns of behavior in reponse to meeting the needs of unconscious drives. Thus, Freud's contribution of explaining mental illnesses as stemming from internal sources complemented Claude Bernard's biological explanation of the internal environment and allowed for the evolution of what might today be called a unitary concept of disease.

Alexis Carrel (1935), the Nobel laureate surgeon and a researcher at the Rockefeller University for many years, believed that medical knowledge should entail the psychological components that Freud pioneered. He describes his view of the support of this unitary concept:

> The physician must clearly distinguish the sick human being described in his books from the concrete patient whom he has to treat, who must not only be studied, but above all, relieved, encouraged, and cured . . . . *His role* is to discover the characteristics of the sick man's individuality, his resistance to pathogenic factors, his sensibility to pain, the value of his organic activities, his past and his future. The outcome of an illness in a given individual has to be predicted, not by a calculation of the probabilities, but by precise analysis of the organic, humoral and psychological personality of this individual. In fact, medicine, when confining itself to the study of diseases, amputates a part of its own body.

Dr. Stewart Wolf (1976), one of the eminent medical minds who pioneered work in demonstrating connections between states of illness and thought processes, also calls for a more unified approach: "Investigations at the molecular, cellular and tissue level that have contributed so much to the rapid progress of our understanding must now give way to a greater emphasis on studies at the organismal level, studies of the whole conscious behaving organism, preferably man."

Dr. Lauro Halstead (1978), associate professor at Baylor College of Medicine, prepared an interesting comparison of scientific (reductionist) and humanistic (holistic) medicine, selecting a number of elements in the health care system. He uses extremes to illustrate his point more clearly, although he calls for a balance of the two approaches. I think these approaches effectively summarize what we have been describing.

1. PROBLEM ORIENTATION: The orientation of scientific medicine is toward disease, while the orientation of humanistic medicine is toward illness. Disease is essentially a biologic event. Illness, on the other hand, is essentially a human event.

2. PHYSICIAN'S ROLE: In scientific medicine, the physician's role tends to be active. The humanistic physician is closer to the original meaning of doctor as teacher.

3. PATIENT'S ROLE: In a scientific setting, the patient's role is often passive; diagnostic and therapeutic measures are done or given to him. By contrast, in humanistic medicine, the patient is encouraged to be an active, informed participant.

4. PHYSICIAN'S RELATION TO PATIENT: In scientific medicine, the physician's relation to the patient is detached, reserved, impersonal; while in humanistic medicine, it is emphatic, personal, close.

5. PHYSICIAN'S RELATION TO HEALTH TEAM: In a scientific setting, health care teams are hierarchical, and the physician, if not dominant, is more equal than other members: in a humanistic approach, the team is egalitarian and the physician is facilitative.

6. PHYSICIAN'S RELATION TO COLLEAGUES: In a scientific approach, a physician's relations to colleagues is characterized by being competitive: while in a humanistic approach, physicians are supportive and collaborative.

7. THERAPEUTIC APPROACH: The therapeutic emphasis in scientific medicine is on treatment; while in humanistic medicine, it is on management. Treatment is defined as effecting a relief or cure of a disease and relies heavily on medication, surgery, and the skills of modern technology. Management, on the other hand, is defined as effecting relief from an illness and enhancing function using the full resources

of the health care system. It implies long-term involvement that actively includes the patient and his family.

I would view the effective blending of these approaches as a call for unified medicine: We need to study the pathogens and their effects on people, as well as the people who are affecting the behavior of the pathogens. Man is more than just a body. He is a mind that thinks thoughts and influences the delicate mechanism of his biochemical and physiologic functions. He is related to all other living things in the universe; he has a purpose beyond just surviving. He is part of a higher, cosmic spiritual force. Unified medicine is more interested in the life-style of the person than just in the lab report; unified medicine spends time to find out about the stress in the person's life that may indicate a belief system that can be damaging and cause disharmony and dis-ease. The sick person is seen as a functioning person instead of a condition.

Unified medicine operates on right-brain intuitive sense (in medical circles, this is known as clinical sense), a faculty of getting some kind of inner direction about what is disrupting the harmony of the patient. It involves a kind of "tuning in" to what is going on. It accepts that germs are agents of disease but, more importantly, it recognizes that stress is the real basis of illness, because stress is the response each individual chooses, consciously or unconsciously, to adapt to internal or external threats. Unified medicine believes that perception of the world is an individual matter that varies from one person to another, thus explaining why each of us sees the world differently.

It is true that the germ theory explains outside factors that are challenges to our adaptation. And the germ theory can be extended to include other "toxins," such as toxic ideas— whether they are social, political, or economic. However, if such outside influences were the determinants of our behavior and our health, it would mean that we possess no personal identity but rather that we are validated by the others in our lives. Our thoughts, our accomplishments, would all be deter- mined by the outside forces that cause us to behave as we do. In a sense, we would see ourselves as victims being acted upon.

How many of us are prepared to accept this explanation of what guides our lives? When we believe that what someone says or does causes our problem or unhappiness, or that pathogenic thoughts and actions in others are threatening to our equilibrium, we begin to act cautiously, and we are suspicious and wary of others, since we conclude that our problems come from their actions. Then we look for ways to defend ourselves or to attack others in order to protect our interest.

The time seems ripe, then, to ask: *Do we intervene to destroy pathogenic agents, or should we work instead to strengthen the person's inherent ability to overcome those agents?* How we answer that question will determine whether we continue in the present model of disease, illness, and pathology, or whether we refocus our attention and energy on a more effective model of health.

In my opinion, one of the greatest single contributions to world medicine and to our understanding of the cause of disease is the monumental work performed by Dr. Hans Selye. His concentrated attention, intuitive insights, and careful observations led to the development of the theory of stress as a basis of illness, a theory that ranks with Pasteur's germ theory and Bernard's interior milieu in scientific importance. We have not yet fully comprehended the significance of Dr. Selye's work, but it is my expectation that as you read the various chapters, the full import of the role of stress in our lives will become apparent.

More and more each day, we are becoming aware of the all-pervasive influence stress plays in our lives. It has become associated with ulcers, asthma, glaucoma, hypertension, cardiovascular problems, diabetes, cancer, arthritis, rheumatism, and allergies, to name a few disorders. As Stewart Wolf (1976) put it: ". . . The length of the list . . . varies with the bias of the author."

Dr. George Engel (1962), one of the most thought-provoking men in medicine today, believes that stress, "directly or indirectly, determines not only the individual's capacity to cope with other stresses but often his exposure to such stresses as well. If these influences are to be clarified, understood and brought under control, medicine must now turn its attention to the central mediating and controlling systems, the brain and the mind."

Nobel Laureate Nikolaas Tinbergen (1974) adds: "It is stress in the widest sense, the inadequacy of our adjustability, that will become perhaps the most important disruptive influence in our society."

Stress is a multi-faceted kind of response that is influenced by a vast array of experiences, thoughts, fears, and attitudes. In short, it is determined by our past experience, in how we perceive or look at the world about us. A given telephone ring can cause pain in the stomach of one person, anger in another, indifference in a third, and eager anticipation and joy in a fourth. All these responses are related to the way each person interprets what that telephone ring means to him. A criticism from the boss can stimulate the heart to race at a dangerous speed in one person, cause muscles to tense in the neck and shoulders of another, stimulate the stomach to secrete large amounts of corrosive hydrochloric acid in a third, and produce a throbbing headache in a fourth.

Different reactions to the same stress factors, such as telephone rings and outside criticism, are obviously determined by our mental programming. They are a product of how we see the world and how we think we are threatened by it. To me, therefore, it would make far more sense to examine and reverse the negative ways we perceive the world than to spend time and money concocting new pills for the relief of distress. Pills give relief, but they only postpone cure. Cure comes from reversing our perceptions, from discovering how we create our own "realities."

Our reactions are most often split second simultaneous responses unconsciously arrived at to produce behavior that most often fits what we have decided, internally, to see first; then, we proceed to see it. It is this *response-ability* which all of us possess and use to keep our world intact as we understand it.

Dr. Jerome Frank (1973), formerly Chairman of the Department of Psychiatry at Johns Hopkins University Medical School, agrees: "Persons differ greatly in the amount of stress they can tolerate; an event that constitutes a crisis for a schizophrenic, for example, might be shrugged off as a minor irritation by a business executive. Furthermore . . . the severity of the stress depends on the meaning of the event to the person, which, in turn, is largely determined by his own life experience. To make matters more complicated, . . . the environmental stress may be largely created by his own behavior."

There is one caution we should exercise in our understanding of the stress response. We may have a tendency to consider it another outside pathogen that once again causes us to submit. There are already signs that this may be happening. We talk about the stress produced by our jobs, our home, our family, our business, the weather, the government, world conditions, and so on. Once again, we are led to believe that we are victims of some outside force that is imposing its will on us and causing dis-stress. "If only my boss would be more understanding," or, "If only we had a Republican president," or, "If only my children would listen to me and behave," and on and on. We produce our own psychological pathogens of stress by the way we choose to perceive and interpret events in our lives. We wait for things outside us to change; then, we think, things will get better.

"When it's warmer weather, I'll feel better and get out."

"When the kids grow up, I'll have more freedom for myself."

"When I get my promotion, my money problem will be solved."

Some people wait all their lives for the outside to change their inside. But it never seems to happen, because change comes from within us first—then the outside becomes different.

I am convinced that we can change our reality by changing how we perceive it, just as beavers build dams and change the course of streams. An enormous amount of work done in the field of hypnosis verifies beyond anyone's doubts that when the conscious perceptive field is temporarily set aside, one then becomes narrowly focused, and all sorts of body responses can be produced merely by suggesting the responses.

A story related to me by my friend Dr. William Thetford, a professor of psychology, is the classical example of the power of suggestion. In his research with volunteers, Dr. Thetford would suggest to them that a hot iron was coming into contact with a spot on their arm. Soon after, a blister would appear on the very spot.

It is important to realize that freedom rests within each human being to choose the way he or she will perceive the world, internally and externally. We can no longer be fooled into thinking that outside forces control our destiny, rule our life, make us sick, or create our reality. We are able to assume the responsibility that the power which created thoughts producing disharmony and disequilibrium is a neutral force that will manifest itself in a form expressed and invented by ourselves and is the same power that can be used to create harmony and balance. (That power is like electricity, also a neutral force, that does not care whether it flows into a vacuum cleaner, a t.v. set, or a piece of laboratory equipment. Electricity is a force that goes where it is directed to flow.) If we are able to help individuals reappraise certain important beliefs about themselves and their self-images, then we are coming to the heart of the basic causes of illness, and we may help to change the course of individual and societal health consciousness.

If it is evident, as I think it is, that the ultimate determinant of how we respond is the way we think, and if this affects the way we feel, we are left with the conclusion that self-regulation of our thoughts is clearly the most likely area to devote our energies toward in health care.

The model of stress reduction developed in this book is not a new one, but it does provide room for all dimensions of our human explorations to find their place and for us to realize that each part of the whole is another way of describing and explaining the same thing. Perhaps we could then begin to look for common denominators that connect branches of science and human endeavors, rather than being conscious of the separation and the differences.

This model fits in with the general direction of holistic health concepts and, thus, prescribes different approaches to the practice of healing. It no longer becomes important as to which modality, specialty, or profession is responsible for the remission of a patient's illness or for the change in significant portions of a lifestyle. Rather, there is a more fundamental role for physicians—as teachers or guides—toward better self-care, working together with other professionals to encourage, as much as possible, the individual's healing capabilities and to maximize their effects.

The remaining chapters of this book will demonstrate how such ideas for the understanding and handling of stress are applied in the physical, mental, and spiritual aspects of man's functioning.

2

Stress: The Basis of Illness

HANS SELYE, PH.D., M.D., D.SC.

It would be instructive to start this chapter by discussing in broad terms the concepts of health, stress, and disease, because patients and doctors, in fact, society as a whole, should be made more aware of the root cause of the medical problems of our times.

If we look at the basic unit of life, the individual cell, we see that it is healthiest when all its parts or constituents are functioning properly and in balance with one another. Higher up in the hierarchy of life, the plant, animal, or human form is likewise healthiest when its various components are well integrated. Thus, on all levels, from the simple unicellular organism to complex human beings and even to entire societies, health is largely determined by stable balance, what Walter Cannon (1939) called homeostasis. Only when parts of the whole function in harmony is the health of the whole assured. Disrupt that balance, and "dis-ease" sets in.

Innumerable studies of disease processes have shown that stress, more than any other factor, determines whether there is a proper balance in our lives. Most of us are born healthy, but if the harmful stresses resulting from improper perception, personal misbehavior, and environmental conditions tip the balance, we slide down the slope from health to disease.

There can be no doubt that stress diseases are on the increase. Cardiac maladies, gastrointestinal disturbances, mental disorders, all stress-induced, are striking people down in their thirties, forties, and early fifties. The tremendous surge of medical progress in recent years has not brought with it any significant improvement in human health. True, we have succeeded in eradicating or at least controlling most of the contagious and infectious diseases, but too much attention has been given to treatment after the fact, to intervention after disease has occurred, rather than to prevention. The past 500 years of medical research have increased our understanding of disease processes, and major advances have been made in the various specialties of medicine, such as anatomy, physiology, pathology, biochemistry, and so on. Now, more than ever before, the great challenge to medicine will be prevention rather than cure. A vast number of people are now desperately searching for protection against disease through self-education, psychotherapeutic techniques, the wisdom of the East, and so on—the list goes on and on. Some succeed in their efforts, but many do not. Beneath all this, we find that there is a common denominator—stress.

Nowadays, the skills and knowledge demanded by any job, as indeed the goals of society itself, are developing or at least changing at such an unprecedented rate that our first objective must be to learn how to cope with the stress of adaptation to change as such, both in our work and in our social goals. Only thus can we hope to succeed in overcoming the distressing loss of stability and perhaps even to enjoy the challenge of adjustment to ever-changing tasks, aspirations, and possibilities.

Of course, the need to adjust to constant change arises from the fact that the more we know and the larger the number of people who acquire knowledge becomes, the faster the pace of development, or at least of exploratory change, becomes in all fields. This situation is primarily created by recent progress in mathematics, physics, chemistry, and engineering, with its resulting industrial implications: computers, automation, and extraordinary acceleration in the rate at which people and information travel and alter the world.

All this is endurable and sometimes even enjoyable, but only within the limits of human adaptability. In the final analysis, the mastery we gain over our inanimate surroundings and the psychosocial consequences thereof are essentially physiologic and medical problems.

For the reasons just mentioned, interest in stress as it influences the lives of individuals and even of entire societies has grown enormously during the past few decades. There has been a phenomenal increase in the number of laboratories, technical articles, books, journals, and congresses dealing with the far-reaching implications of stress in virtually all fields of human endeavor, including medicine, physiology, psychology, psychiatry, sociology, and philosophy. Nowadays, even the lay press, television, and radio are constantly discussing stress, although frequently without real awareness of the objective scientific proofs upon which certain conclusions are based.

The magnitude and danger of the resulting confusion stem mainly from the fact that, unlike all other research subjects, stress (as defined in medicine) affects every aspect of life in health and disease. Indeed, it exerts an ever-increasing influence upon even the most sophisticated activities of the mind. A real understanding of stress is therefore essentially dependent upon a holistic and integrative approach. No special aspect of it can be analyzed in depth without a full realization of where and how it fits into the whole picture of life. On the individual's level, such a better understanding of stress will rightly focus on health, on the prevention of disorders caused by stress, instead of concentrating on treatment after the disorders occur.

DEFINITION OF STRESS

Stress is the nonspecific response of the body to any demand.
It is inherent in all forms of animate (and inanimate) activity.
Therefore, it could not and should not be avoided, for complete
freedom from stress is death.

Just staying alive creates demands on the body for life-
maintaining energy. Even while we sleep, our heart, lungs,
digestive tract, nervous system, and other vital organs must
continue to function. Thus, energy utilization is the foremost
characteristic of biologic stress. In machines, stress manifests
itself in either constructive or destructive activity, and here,
too, energy utilization is the most important, vital requirement.

The second characteristic feature of stress is its nonspeci-
ficity. Any demands made upon us in everyday life elicit certain
reactions in the body. The basic pattern of these reactions is
stereotyped, and it will occur under the most diverse conditions, such as cold, heat, sorrow, joy, and so on. The nature of
the demand is immaterial, because the stress response is always
the same.

Joy, suffering, and physical exhaustion make certain common demands upon us; we must adapt ourselves to something
new. Various mechanisms will trigger nonspecific reactions in
the body under these conditions. Nervous signals are sent from
the brain to several glands, and these react by secreting hormones to cope with the task ahead of us—namely, the demands
being made by the mental or muscular readjustments.

These examples also show the close interrelation of mind
and body in coping with stress-producing situations. The train
of reactions, starting with the hypothalamus and its nervous
signals and ending with the consequent hormonal and muscular
changes, demonstrates the intricate ties that exist between the
mental and physical components of the body.

In the long run, therefore, human adaptation contributes
to the harmony or disharmony of functions and structural
integrity, not only of organs and parts, not only of cells and

their minute components, but also of the organism as a whole in terms of body, mind, and spirit. Thus, although common demands are made for adaptation, the response, though stereotyped, can vary and produce positive benefits or only deleterious effects, depending upon the state of the organism at that point in time.

THE FIGHT OR FLIGHT REACTION

Needless to say, the stress response is an extremely complex phenomenon. Our understanding of it was made possible through countless animal experiments performed all over the world, starting perhaps with Walter Cannon's classic investigations in cats and dogs (1939).

Cannon proved that higher animal species defend themselves against various types of aggression, insult, or injury by a single fundamental response, which he called the "fight or flight" response. He showed that challenges to the animal's normal resting equilibrium were met by this stereotypical reaction that varied in intensity with the force of the stressor agent. The reaction, he theorized, was built into the animal's defense system as a safety measure in order to ensure its survival.

This basic defense reaction pattern in animals and even in man has not yet been fully clarified. It took millions of years of evolution for Nature to gradually work out the best possible defense for survival. Hence, we can reasonably assume that it will take many more years before we can dissect the complicated network of interacting events that are triggered by confrontation with a stressor.

PATHWAYS MEDIATING THE STRESS RESPONSE

We still do not know how a nonspecific stimulus is produced by a stressor acting upon the body, except that something must convey the message from the directly affected region to the centers of adaptation that a state of stress exists. This first effect could be a nervous impulse, a chemical substance, or even the depletion of an indispensable metabolic factor. We simply call it the "first mediator," because nothing is known about its nature. We cannot even be certain that it is an excess or a deficiency of a particular substance. Man is endowed with a highly developed nervous system, and, hence, the stress response could well be initiated by emotional arousal. But stress reactions also occur in plants and in lower animals that have no nervous systems. Furthermore, patients under deep anesthesia show typical stress responses to such stressors as trauma, hemorrhage, and so on. Thus, it can be seen that conscious psychic disturbances are not indispensable in order for typical somatic stress reactions to occur. It is tempting to speculate at this point that cell consciousness is common to all life forms and that cells respond to stressors, always with the purpose of re-establishing the homeostatic balance or equilibrium.

Hormonal Mechanisms

Although the "first mediator" has still to be identified, we do know that, at least in man and other mammals, eventually the stressor excites the hypothalamus, a complex bundle of nerve cells and fibers that acts as a bridge between the brain and the endocrine system (Selye, 1976). The message is relayed to the first endocrine gland in this chain, the pituitary, and the result is a discharge of ACTH (*a*dreno*c*ortico*t*rophic *h*ormone) from the pituitary into the general circulation. Upon reaching the adrenal cortex, ACTH triggers the secretion of corticoids, mainly glucocorticoids, such as cortisol or corticosterone. These "stress hormones" supply a readily available source of energy for the adaptive reactions necessary to meet the demands made by the stressor agent. The corticoids also facilitate various other enzyme responses, and they suppress immune reactions as well as inflammation, thereby helping the body to coexist with potential pathogens. This complex chain of events is cybernetically controlled by several feedback mechanisms (see Figure 2–1). As soon as any agent acts upon the body (thick outer frame of the diagram), the resulting effect will depend upon three factors: stressor agents and internal and external conditioning. All agents possess both nonspecific stressor effects (solid part of arrow) and specific properties (interrupted part of arrow). The latter vary with each individual agent; they are inseparably attached to the stressor effect and invariably modify it. Two arrows represent the exogenous and endogenous conditioning factors which largely determine the reactivity of the body. Since all stressors have some specific effects, they cannot elicit exactly the same response in all organs. Furthermore, even the same agent will act differently in different individuals, depending upon the internal and external conditioning factors which determine their reactivity.

At the same time as these events are taking place, another important pathway is utilized to mediate the stress response. Other stress hormones, such as catecholamines, are liberated, and they activate mechanisms of general utility to meet the various demands for adaptation. Epinephrine or adrenalin in particular is secreted to provide energy, to accelerate the pulse rate, to elevate blood pressure, and to quicken blood circulation in the muscles, as well as to stimulate the central nervous system. The blood coagulation mechanism is also activated, and this protects against excessive bleeding if injuries are sustained in the encounter with the stressor. All these coping measures help the organism in its "fight or flight" response (Selye, 1976).

This brief and simplified description of the stress reaction is by no means complete. Innumerable other hormonal and chemical changes check and balance the body's functioning and stability. They represent a virtual arsenal of weapons by which the organism defends itself for survival.

One of the most characteristic features of all living beings is their ability to maintain the constancy of their internal milieu, despite changes in the surroundings. The physical properties and chemical composition of our body fluids and tissues tend to remain remarkably constant despite all the changes around us. For instance, if we are exposed to extreme

Figure 2.1 Principal pathways mediating the response to a stressor agent and the conditioning factors that modify its effect. (Printed with courtesy of Butterworths, Reading, Mass., from H. Selye, *Stress in Health and Disease,* 1976.)

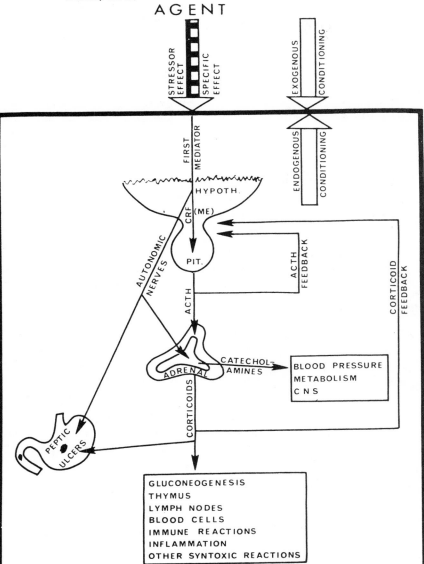

cold or heat, our bodies will try to maintain a constant temperature. If this self-regulatory power fails, disease or even death will ensue. Homeostasis, the staying power of the body in an ever-changing environment, is therefore the all-important criterion of health.

Nervous Mechanisms

The hypothalamus functions through the two divisions of the autonomic nervous system: the sympathetic and parasympathetic nerves. In addition to regulating growth, sex, and reproduction, it is responsible for stimulating the emotions of fear, rage, and pleasure, to name a few. The sympathetic system passes through the spinal cord to specific organs through large ganglia or nerve clusters. The functions of this system manifest themselves in muscular movements of the stomach, intestine, and bladder. Face muscles contract or contort under the influence of the emotions. The pupils dilate, the nostrils flare, and the throat passage widens. Breathing becomes fast, raising the pulse rate and carrying extra oxygen to vital areas. Digestion by the stomach and intestine is temporarily suspended. The muscles controlling the bowels and bladder become loose. These are some of the physiologic features of the "fight or flight" reaction.

The body is now mobilized for action. There is evidently increased strength and vigor because digestion has stopped along with other functions that are not needed for fight or flight. Now, the accelerated clotting time will heal wounds rapidly, and the proliferation of white blood cells will counteract infection. Perspiration cools the entire organism through the evaporation of sweat, and bodily wastes are eliminated as well.

All these phenomena again demonstrate that there is a close integration of mind and body. Much more detailed scientific investigation would be needed before we could arrive at a comprehensive and systematic analysis of the separate adaptive phenomena indispensable for the maintenance of life under special conditions.

If we are to attempt a detailed discussion of stress, we must also take into consideration those first basic animal experiments performed to dissect the mechanisms of stress, since these investigations are at the very basis of stress research in the world today.

PHYSIOLOGIC MANIFESTATIONS OF STRESS

In the late 1930s, to establish the evolution of the stress response, we had to expose rats repeatedly to such extreme stressors as cold, forced muscular exercise, bone fracture, and so on. These stress-producing agents (stressors) were of a constant intensity, and they made demands for adaptation over long periods of time (Selye, 1956).

It gradually turned out that no matter what type of damage was inflicted upon the rats, if they survived long enough and if the stressor was sufficiently strong, a characteristic triad of symptoms was produced:

1. The adrenal cortex became enlarged.
2. The thymus, spleen, lymph nodes, and all other lymphatic structures showed severe involution.
3. Deep bleeding ulcers appeared in the stomach and duodenum.

Thus, adrenal enlargement, thymicolymphatic involution, and gastrointestinal ulcers seemed to be the omnipresent signs of damage to the body when under attack (see Figure 2–2). In the typical triad of the alarm reaction, the adrenals of the alarmed rat (*right*) are obviously enlarged; there is, in addition, loss of whitish corticoid-laden lipids and hyperemia of the adrenals, which consequently become reddish brown. The thymus and lymph nodes show intense atrophy, and the gastric mucosa is spotted with numerous blood-covered ulcers.

When the body shows the changes characteristic of the first exposure to a stressor, initially, in the alarm reaction, the

Figure 2.2 The typical triad of the alarm reaction. (Reprinted with permission from Selye, *The Story of the Adaptation Syndrome.* Courtesy Acta, Inc., Montreal, 1952).

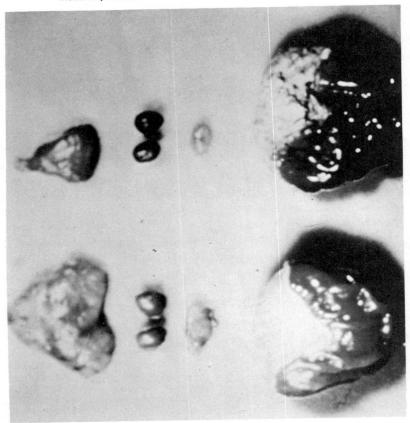

body's resistance is diminished (Figure 2–3) and, if the stressor is sufficiently strong (severe burns, extremes of temperature, etc.), death may result. Resistance ensues if continued exposure to the stressor is compatible with adaptation. The bodily signs characteristic of the alarm reaction have virtually disappeared, and resistance rises above normal. Following long, continued exposure to the same stressor, to which the body has become adjusted, eventually adaptation energy is exhausted. The signs of the alarm reaction reappear, but now they are irreversible, and the individual dies. This was borne out in further studies. We demonstrated that this syndrome evolved in three stages: the alarm reaction, the stage of resistance, and the stage of exhaustion. Apparently, just like the resources of this planet, the adaptation energy of all living organisms is not unlimited but finite.

Figure 2.3 The three phases of the General Adaptation Syndrome. (Printed with courtesy of J. B. Lippincott from *Stress Without Distress,* 1974.)

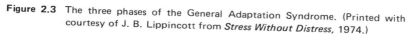

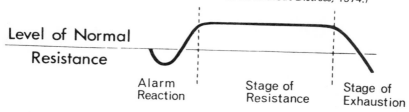

The initial exposure to the stressor produced the nonspecific response characterized by the triad of adrenal enlargement, thymicolymphatic involution, and gastrointestinal ulcers. This first stage, which we called the alarm reaction, represented a generalized call to arms of the body's defensive forces. In other words, the rat seemed to be preparing itself for "fight or flight." It then passed into the second phase, the stage of resistance.

The rat became adapted to the challenge and even began to resist it. The length of this stage of resistance depended, of course, on the body's innate adaptation energy and on the intensity of the stressor. The chemical changes were the exact opposite of those observed during the alarm reaction.

But just as any inanimate machine gradually wears out, even if it has enough fuel, so does the living organism sooner or later become the victim of constant wear and tear. The acquired adaptation is lost if the animal is subjected to still more exposure to the stressor. It enters the third and final stage: the stage of exhaustion. And then it dies. It has used up its fund of "adaptation energy" (see Figure 2-3).

The triphasic response of the general adaptation syndrome

(G.A.S.) gave us the first indication that the body's adaptability is finite. It is tempting to view the G.A.S. as a kind of accelerated aging. It appears as though, because of the greater intensity of stress, the three major periods of life—infancy (in which adaptation has not yet been acquired), adulthood (in which adaptation has developed to meet the usual stresses of life), and senility (in which the acquired adaptation is lost again)—are here telescoped into a short space of time (Selye, 1974).

Every part of the body is involved in the stress response, but the two great integrators of activity, the hormonal and the nervous systems, are especially important. The facts known today lead us to believe that the anterior pituitary and the adrenal cortex play cardinal roles in coordinating the defense of the organism during stress. This view is probably distorted because the G.A.S. has been studied primarily by endocrinologists, and because investigations concerning the participation of the nervous system are handicapped by the greater complexity of the required techniques.

Even so, the advances made by such "specialized approaches," the development of new methodologies, and the progress achieved in identifying individual mechanisms, whether hormonal or nervous, should not cloud our vision of the organism as an interacting whole, an organism whose internal functions and parts must necessarily perform in harmony, an organism that is also in balance with the myriad forces of the external environment.

CONDITIONING FACTORS

We must not forget that the stress response is also largely influenced by heredity, age, previous exposure to stress, nervous stimuli, the nutritional state of the organism, and many other factors. All these conditioners alter the production of adaptive hormones, and, consequently, the stressor effect modifies the entire state of the body. Perhaps the most significant, and therefore the most important, consideration here is the way each individual views or "perceives" a given situation, based on his needs, aspirations, and past experiences. Therefore, the stress accruing from that situation will be determined largely by how he "interprets" it, conditioned as he is by his fears, anxieties, and frustrations.

Under the influence of such internal or external (endogenous or exogenous) conditioning factors, a normally well-tolerated degree of stress can but does not necessarily become pathogenic and cause diseases of adaptation. It might or might not selectively affect those parts of the body that are particularly sensitized, both by the conditioning factors and by the specific effect of the stressor agent. This selectivity of damage is comparable to that in different chains, in each of which, mechanical stress of identical tension will break the particular link that has become weakest as a result of internal or external factors.

DISEASES OF ADAPTATION

Under certain circumstances, animals in a state of severe stress develop diseases which we have called "stress diseases" or "diseases of adaptation"—for example, hardening of the arteries, kidney disorders, severe bleeding peptic ulcers, physiologic changes reminiscent of arthritis, and other maladies closely resembling those that tend to occur as a consequence of constant, intense stress (heart accidents, mental exhaustion, and so on). It is clear that many of these diseases are the result of improper functioning of the pituitary and adrenals during emergencies arising from demands for adaptation to changing circumstances.

These same phenomena can be observed every day all around us. For years, most of us resist the stresses caused by preoccupations, frustrations, physical fatigue, tension, overwork, cigarette smoking, excessive alcohol consumption, chronic infections, and innumerable other agents that demand constant adaptation. Finally, however, there comes a day when a normally well-balanced person begins to show signs of increased blood pressure, suffers a heart attack, or notices the signs of a gastrointestinal peptic ulcer (Blythe, 1973; Wolf and Goodell, 1968).

By "diseases of adaptation," we mean maladies that are caused principally by errors in the general adaptation process. The pathogenicity of many systemic and local stressors depends largely upon the function of the hypothalamus-pituitary-adrenal axis. The latter may either enhance or mitigate the body's defense reactions against stressors. We think that derailments of this adaptive mechanism are the principal factors in the production of certain maladies, which we therefore consider to be essentially "diseases of adaptation."

However, we should not assume that stress diseases are inevitable. They will not occur when all the regulatory processes are properly checked and balanced. They will not develop when adaptation is facilitated by improved perception and interpretation. Thus, adaptation need not necessarily result in disease, for the toll it exacts will ultimately depend upon how we see our world as individuals.

Among the derailments of the G.A.S. that may cause disease, perhaps the most important is an absolute excess, deficiency, or disequilibrium in the amount of adaptive hormones—for example, corticoids, ACTH, and growth hormone—produced during stress.

But although it is true that the hypothalamus-pituitary-adrenal mechanism plays a prominent role in the G.A.S., other organs that participate in the latter (for example, the nervous system, the liver, and the kidney) may also respond abnormally and become the cause of disease during adaptation to stress.

This cause and effect relationship is necessarily simplified for an understanding of the mechanisms of stress. It does not follow that we fully comprehend the stress-and-disease process, because the tendency is to give too much importance to particular diseased organs, failing to be sufficiently aware of the relationship of many other organ systems that will be affected by stress. Indeed, it should be emphasized that disease usually manifests itself only in those organs that are most prominently disturbed. Sometimes, dysfunction of a given organ may even surface as perturbations in another, far-removed site.

With all this in mind, it may be convenient for investigative purposes to classify as "diseases of adaptation" those maladies in which an inadequacy of the adaptation syndrome plays a particularly important role. This means that the term should be used only when the maladaptation factor appears to be more important than the eliciting pathogen itself. No disease is purely a disease of adaptation, any more than it could be purely a disease of the heart or an infectious disease in which adaptive phenomena play no part.

In any event, in addition to studying disease processes, we need to give considerably more attention to the mechanisms behind the adaptation syndrome and to the selective measures that the individual uses in coping with stress. Too much consideration has been directed towards specific pathogens and towards specific disease models, and not enough consideration has been given to the patient and to how he developed his particular disease. It is being said with increasing force and frequency that we must shift our focus from diseased parts to the whole being, for only then can we learn more about what activates the adaptation syndrome at all levels within the organism. Only then can we understand why stress affects different people in different ways.

ANIMAL EXPERIMENTS AND THEIR CLINICAL IMPLICATIONS

Since most of the fundamental work on stress has been performed on laboratory animals, it was reasonable to question its applicability to problems of health and clinical medicine. It may now be said, however, that although there are certain differences in the stress response of every species, the general pattern of physiologic reactions is essentially the same in the various kinds of experimental animals and in man. Furthermore, a good deal of evidence has accumulated in support of the view that the experimental similes of spontaneous diseases produced in animals, either by exposure to stress or by overdosage with certain adaptive hormones, are closely related to the corresponding maladies of man.

Let us merely mention a few of the striking similarities in the responses to stress and to adaptive hormones in animals and man.

Physiologic Effects of Adaptive Hormones

There can be no doubt that, during intense stress (for example, severe mechanical or thermal injuries and massive infections), the adrenal cortex of man, like that of laboratory animals, shows morphologic changes characteristic of hyperactivity. At the same time, there is a demonstrable increase in the blood concentration and urinary excretion of corticoids and their metabolites. The other manifestations (morphologic, functional, and chemical) of the stress syndrome also fail to exhibit any fundamental dissimilarity in the reaction patterns of animals and man (Selye, 1970; 1971).

During stress, the corticoid requirements of all mammals are far above normal. After destruction of the adrenals by disease (as after their surgical removal), the daily dose of corticoids necessary for the maintenance of well-being at rest is comparatively small, but it rises sharply during stress (for example, cold, recurrent infections, and hemorrhage), both in experimental animals and in man.

The same antiphlogistic corticoids (for example, cortisone and cortisol) that inhibit various types of experimental inflammations in laboratory animals exert similar effects in a human being afflicted by inflammatory diseases (for example, rheumatoid arthritis, rheumatic fever, and allergic inflammations).

In experimental animals, the suppression of inflammation by antiphlogistic hormones is frequently accompanied by an increased sensitivity to infection, presumably because the encapsulation of microbial foci is less effective, and perhaps also partly because serologic defense is diminished. Thus, even a species naturally resistant to the human type of tuberculosis, such as the rat, can contract this disease during overdosage with ACTH or cortisone (see Figure 2-4). The rat, naturally resistant to tuberculosis, normally shows no response. After destruction of its defensive abilities, it dies with widespread tuberculosis. Similarly, in patients undergoing intense treatment with antiphlogistic hormones (for example, for rheumatoid arthritis), a previously latent tuberculous focus may suddenly spread. It is a well-known fact that in patients suffering from tuberculosis, the disease is especially readily aggravated by exposure to any kind of stress situation. Rest cures have therefore long been advocated. It is perhaps not too far-fetched to consider the possibility that an increased ACTH and cortisol secretion during stress may play an important part in the development of clinical tuberculosis.

Psychologic Effects of Adaptive Hormones

Considerable attention has been given of late to the possible mental effects of stress and of the adaptive hormones. It would be beyond the scope of this chapter to discuss these findings

Figure 2.4 Low magnification of lungs of rats.

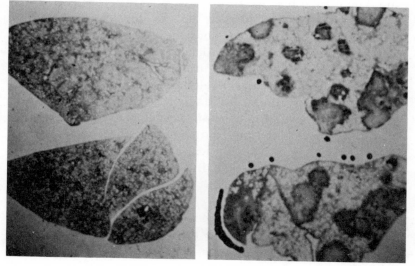

in detail, but a few remarks based on our experimental observations may be in order to underscore the close interrelation of the somatic and psychic components of man.

It has long been noted that various steroids—including desoxycorticosterone, cortisone, progesterone, and many others—can produce in a variety of animal species (even in primates such as the rhesus monkey) a state of great excitation followed by deep anesthesia (Selye, 1971). It has more recently been shown that such steroid anesthesia can also be produced in man, and, of course, the marked emotional changes (sometimes bordering on psychosis) that may occur in predisposed individuals during treatment with ACTH, cortisone, and cortisol are well known. Furthermore, several laboratories have reported that the electroshock threshold of experimental animals and their sensitivity to anesthetics can be affected by corticoids.

Thus, it appears very probable that corticoids secreted during stress also have an important influence on nervous and emotional reactions. Conversely, it is now definitely established that nervous stressors (pain and emotions) are particularly conducive to the development of the somatic manifestations of the stress syndrome. Thus, stress can both cause and be caused by mental reactions.

We should also re-emphasize that no illness is exclusively a disease of adaptation; but considerable evidence has accumulated in favor of the view that stress, and particularly the adaptive hormones produced during stress, exert an important regulating influence on the development of numerous maladies.

All these observations and findings in laboratories throughout the world have only confirmed what man has known subconsciously since time immemorial. Pre-civilized man felt the stresses of hunger, cold, physical fatigue, and so on just as does his contemporary today. But the tensions and strains of his daily existence were much less complicated and far less insidious.

Today's medical practice, at least as we know it in the West, has only just started to explore the close interrelation of body and mind. Science as such has not been able to clarify the nature of man, although it has been well established that "man's ability to adapt in order to remain free of illness depends not only on his own inherent capacities and past experience, but also on his motivation and the support and refreshment that his environment can afford him" (Wolf and Goodell, 1976). The goal of medicine should therefore be to understand the patient as a person: to establish the circumstances that precipitated his illness—the underlying conflicts, hostilities, and griefs; in short, the bruised nature of his emotional state. The physician needs to know as much about emotions and emotional maladjustments as about disease symptoms and drugs. This approach holds more promise of cure than anything that medicine has given man (Wolf and Goodell, 1976).

THE ANXIETY OF TECHNOLOGY

Man's highly developed brain has produced sophisticated technology, and this knowledge has generated an unprecedented speed and spread of information. He now has to communicate with the teeming multitude around him, and his interrelations are fraught with pleasures, mood changes, threats, and an incredible number of situations and events that cause excessive stress. His interpersonal relations now have more and more pleasant and unpleasant connotations, because he feels the growing need to control events in his life and in his environment. But such control is sometimes beyond the individual's power. He therefore tries to anticipate and to prepare, plan, and act accordingly, and usually anticipation of events proves to be more stressful that the actual events themselves. Some have even called the twentieth century the Age of Anxiety, the Age of Uncertainty, or Future Shock (Albrecht, 1979, Sarason and Spielberger, 1976).

Today's technologic progress or process has advertently or inadvertently reduced the quality of man's life, his food, his environment, and even his behavior—all of which determine health and well-being. Technologic societies—and most societies aspire to reach the highest possible level—are totally committed to economic or industrial growth. Steady state policies rarely exist. The demands created by growth are increasingly far-reaching. They prey on the finite resources of this planet and steer us away from our basic instincts of survival and natural well-being. Somehow, many of us have surrendered our innate responsibilities to others—doctors, hospitals, institutions, the state.

But the tremendous surge in medical progress in recent years has not brought with it any significant improvement in human health. In fact, these awesome advances have tended to cloud our vision of health, and we take it for granted until it is too late. We do not want to live on a "bland regime of health." Moreover, we also tend to assume that institutionalized medicine guarantees us a disease-free existence. The average doctor is today inundated with sick patients, but no one in particular could be faulted for this unhealthy state of affairs. The greatest threat to man seems to be himself and his own kind. "We have met the enemy and it is us" (Knowles, 1977).

In the past, governments all over the world were largely preoccupied with reducing mortality rates, and rightly so. Now, however, increasing attention is being paid also to improving the quality of life by reducing morbidity and enhancing physical, mental and social well-being.

Severely disabling, although not necessarily life-threatening mental and physical disorders are widespread in developing and developed countries alike. So are distress and human suffering. The latter, however, still tend to be accepted as characteristics of human existence to such a degree that possible counter-measures are liable to be disregarded. Although fundamental to most eastern philosophies and to the way of life of preliterate peoples, the "quality of life" concept has been dismissed by many in the industrialized world as vague and devoid of operational content. Yet recent experience of growing dissatisfaction with the conditions of contemporary life indicates that to ignore this aspect is to imperil each of our separate efforts towards meeting human needs.

Quality of life has many aspects. Having ensured the satisfaction of our most immediate needs, we expect a certain amount of security, freedom, equality, belongingness, companionship, information, participation, power and resources. In doing so, we tend to forget that a certain amount of one component often means relinquishing one or several of the others. The good life is a dynamic balance of satisfaction of all these components, a balance which cannot be determined by experts. It will differ from person to person and will characterize each individual. This must be kept in mind so as to design a policy with so much flexibility and freedom of choice that each man is able to arrive at his personal combination. Clearly, we are still very far from this utopian goal (Levi and Andersson, 1975).

Meanwhile, men and women in modern society are wreaking havoc on their physical and mental health and on that of their families and friends. They seem to forget that modern life means great change, and great change is great stress, but it may be good or bad stress. We only need to look at the much-quoted Holmes and Rahe life events scale (Selye, 1976; Tanner, 1976) to realize that the more profound the life change, the greater will be the possibility of stress and illness.

This is not to say that change is unnecessary, for who would want to live a life of "no hits, no runs, no errors." Change could and should be a dynamic force in human growth and development. Its beneficial effects can be fully exploited with heightened self-awareness of individual strengths and weaknesses, capabilities and limitations—all of which are indicators of one's stress level. One should strike for the highest attainable aims but never put up resistance in vain (Selye, 1974).

STRESS—THE SILENT KILLER

Some people are killed in automobile accidents or by other physical forces of destruction, but stress, though an intangible, can kill just as swiftly and surely. Many experts are now claiming that extreme stress can cause cancer in man and animals by suppressing the immune system. Even though there is no conclusive evidence for these claims, the connection cannot be completely ignored. Heart diseases, most due to stressful events and lifestyles, have reached epidemic proportions in the United States, and these disorders seem to be on the rise, along with the American gross national product (Knowles, 1977).

The continuous flooding of our bodies with adaptive hormones also has other not so serious effects, but it should be re-emphasized that once "dis-ease" sets in, permanent if not lethal damage is not too far away. We have demonstrated quite convincingly that certain adaptive hormones lower the rat's resistance and make it susceptible to tuberculosis (see Figure 2-4). It is now becoming increasingly clear that excessive stress affects the immune system, sometimes making the organism highly sensitive to usually harmless microorganisms. As we mentioned earlier, one of the characteristic features of the G.A.S. is thymicolymphatic involution (see Figure 2-2). And, since this system operates the body's immune mechanisms, it is small wonder that if it is damaged in any way, serious immunologic disturbances can be created.

STRESS AND IMMUNITY

Severe stress suppresses inflammation and immune reactions by influencing the defense system. Unfortunately, if chronically induced, this defensive response also lowers the resistance of the organism, since fewer antibodies are produced, and the inflammatory response dwindles. In real life, this diminished resistance makes people hypersensitive to otherwise harmless pollen, to cat or dog hair, to mushrooms, to strawberries, and sometimes even to other people. It is now common knowledge that asthma attacks are elicited, or at least facilitated, by stressful experiences. Stress, in these cases, is more often than not the basis of illness. In fact, we are only now beginning to expand our understanding of psychosomatic medicine. This firmly established science might even lead to another branch, that of somatopsychic medicine (Selye, 1956), because bodily changes can affect mentality just as mental changes can affect the body.

Thus, it is extremely hard to differentiate a disease as being either somatic or psychic, because the interrelation of mind and body is deeper and more complex than we thought it to be. Occasional cancer, for instance, appears to be quite common among seemingly healthy people. However, as long as the immune system is functioning, and functioning efficiently, the growth of such cancers will usually be suppressed. But even a slight shift in cellular balance—that is, a shift in the chemical composition or functionality of cellular components—can produce a malignant growth. It is even claimed that everybody has some cancerous cells but that they are kept in check by a properly functioning immune system. Naturally, if this theory is true, then it would follow that failure of the immune system would produce cancer or some other tumors (Lamott, 1974; McQuade and Aikman, 1974).

Medicine has today progressed to such an extent that the world literature is often conflicting and contradictory. The study of life in hospitals and laboratories does not necessarily give us an accurate picture of the way nature functions. Each of us is unique, an individual, and our problems in health and disease are likewise different. Our genetic make-up, education, environment, and innumerable other factors condition us in different ways. So, we can try to make broad generalizations about cause and effect relationships, but the task is certainly not an easy one.

For instance, Friedman and Rosenman (1974) have correlated Type A behavior with coronary heart disease, and the pioneering work of these investigators is only now beginning to have a widespread effect, especially on business and industry. But their description of Type A and Type B personalities (what we used to call the "stress seekers" and "stress avoiders") gives the impression that these are congenital traits, sort of unchangeable acts of fate. Not quite so. One needs to consider also that "personality" as such is influenced by past experiences and education, that people are largely products of their environment.

But how can we cope with stress? How can we recognize its various forms and shapes? After all, stress is only an abstraction.

True, stress is an abstraction, but so is the wind, electricity, and many other force fields as we know them in physics. Indeed, life itself is an abstraction. No one has succeeded in studying life in a pure, uncontaminated form. It is always inseparably attached to something that lives (i. e., cells, tissue, organs, or other substances that manifest life) which is more tangible and seemingly more real. And the whole science of physiology is built upon this abstraction!

Of course, despite its limited capacities, the unlimited curiosity of the human brain may eventually permit man to solve this or any other fundamental questions. But to begin somewhere, we must clearly realize that stress is a condition, a state of body and mind, and as such it is imponderable; but it manifests itself by measurable chemical changes in the organs of the body. In human beings, stress is largely a matter of perception and interpretation: It is extremely important that we recognize this fact. In the final analysis, aside from their inherent effects *per se*, the actions of stressors are primarily dependent upon "how we take them," upon how we perceive the stimuli and how we react to them as actually being eu-stressful or distressful. This is, or should be, recognized by all of us if we want to know how to cope well with the stress of life today.

CAN WE REALLY COPE WITH STRESS?

It only takes a little reflection and thought to realize that we cannot escape stress caused by awesome technologic changes. The big push from rural to urban areas has altered life dramatically. Dwelling in large apartment houses is nowadays so commonplace that it has become casual, yet, when you come to think of it, such lifestyles did not exist more than a century ago. If we compare this situation with the experiments performed on crowding among rats, we cannot but feel that it will somehow generate behavioral aberrations. Economic factors are dominating our lives, and just getting to work at the office often requires a high level of stress resistance. It has become a truism that crowding and an accelerated pace of life induce almost unremitting arousal within the body.

There seem to be no escape routes for the individual. Many turn to drugs, alcohol, tobacco, coffee, and snacking foods, but these only mask the symptoms of distress. They temporarily displace distress by euphoria or by an artificial feeling of well-being, but few of us realize that these escapes are stressors in themselves and that they add to the overall stress of our lives. Some choose to take the more irreversible avenue of suicide, the incidence of which usually rises at times of emotional strain or economic crisis. We are developing into a generation of "escape artists" and our twentieth-century "fight or flight" reaction is fast becoming a monstrous scientific curiosity. We often mobilize our bodies involuntarily for fight or flight, but we seldom carry through the process in physical terms—we stew in our own juices, so to speak. It should be clear, then, that we need to tune ourselves down, to unwind. If we do not learn the skills to relax and to allow our bodies time and a chance to cure themselves, we will always be living well above our level of stress resistance, well beyond our means—our limited fund of adaptation energy. We must learn how to eliminate low-level anxiety and take things as they come, without perceiving them as exaggerated threats to our well-being. Crises need to be avoided, and we should all accept our responsibilities to ourselves by looking after our health—physical, mental, and spiritual. The integrating concept of body, mind, and spirit is assuming phenomenal popularity and importance. The holistic approach aims at naturally enhancing our total self-awareness and well-being. By learning to gauge our innate energy, our potential weaknesses and strengths, each of us can learn how to improve his or her health and behavior. It requires a great deal of self-discipline and the development of will power.

Above all, we must not lose sight of that vital, innate awareness that each of us is responsible for his or her own health and
well-being. We need to adopt this guiding principle unequivo-
cally, or else we will continue to be plagued by stress-induced
diseases.

It is heartening to witness the now so popular search for
inner awareness through experiential activities and introspec-
tion. This change in course, this altered direction, this increased
consciousness, achieved by thousands through the practice of
the most diverse techniques, holds the answer to mankind's
future and well-being as a life force that must necessarily live
in harmony with itself and with the other myriad life forms
of the environment.

THE CONCEPT OF SPECIFICITY

Pasteur, Koch, and their contemporaries introduced the
concept of specificity into medicine, a concept that has proved
to be of the greatest heuristic value up to the present time. Each
individual, well-defined disease, they held, has its own specific
cause. It has been claimed by many that Pasteur failed to
recognize the importance of the "terrain" because he was too
preoccupied with the pathogen, the microorganism, itself. His
work on induced immunity shows that this is incorrect. Indeed,
at the end of his life, he allegedly said, *"Le microbe n'est rien,
le terrain est tout"* (The microbe is nothing, the terrain is
everything).

The theory that directed the most fruitful investigations of
Pasteur and his followers was that the organism can develop
specific adaptive reactions against individual pathogens and that
by imitating and complementing these, whenever they are
short of optimal, we can treat many of the diseases that are
caused by specific pathogens.

To my mind, the G.A.S. represents, in a sense, the negative

counterpart, or mirror image, of this concept. It holds that many diseases have no single cause, no specific pathogen, but are largely due to nonspecific stress and to pathogenic situations that result from improper perception and/or inappropriate responses to various challenges and demands.

Our understanding of the pathways through which stress acts may be partly incorrect. It is certainly quite incomplete. But what little we know already gives us a basis for the objective scientific dissection of such time-honored, but hitherto rather vague, concepts as the roles of "reactivity" of "constitution," and of "resistance" in the genesis and treatment of disease.

If I may venture a prediction, I would like to reiterate my opinion that research on stress will be most fruitful if it is guided by the principle that we must learn to imitate—and, if necessary, to correct and complement—the body's own auto-pharmacologic efforts to combat the stress factor in our lives.

This new-old view of health and disease, then, is that they are not merely individual interactions between pathogens and human beings but that they involve an entire spectrum of other relationships, including those with one's spouse, employer, children, neighbors, and spiritual or medical advisors.

The questions we must ask ourselves now are philosophical and ethical ones. As John H. Knowles (1977) put it in *Doing Better and Feeling Worse*:

> In its power, then, to change the conditions of birth and death, to alter ways of life and behavior, to impose new dilemmas about the relationship between individual and social good, medical research and clinical practice force a new confrontation with some of the oldest of human questions. What do we account as "happiness," and what should medicine's role be in bringing it about? What is a "good death," and what are the possibilities and limitations of medicine in contributing to that? How much sacrifice of individual health can society demand in the name of general health? How far must society go in making use of medical means to satisfy individual and sometimes idiosyncratic desires?

WHAT IS HEALTH?

Man has always been preoccupied with his health and wanted to improve it, both as regards the mind and the body. Throughout history, innumerable great thinkers have approached the problem from the point of view of theology, psychology, sociology, and, of course, particularly medicine, but whatever the approach or technique they favored, the point of view was always specialized. Only recently, through meetings of such diverse experts as those represented in this book, are we beginning to really look upon health as an holistic problem. After all, we are thinking of the health of man as such, and we will never arrive at a satisfactory solution if all of us take different reductionist points of view. Individually, we are interested in improving health by research limited to molecular biology, electron microscopy, pharmacology, behavioral philosophy (including religious codes), sociology, politics, economics, or any of the other specialized disciplines. But this group of authors, brought together by Dr. Goldwag, has one characteristic feature that, I believe, gives us much hope: Although most, if not all, of us are more or less specialized, we do have an open mind about the holistic approach, and we do not look upon our particular field of expertise as the only all-encompassing solution to man's troubles and the only road to happiness.

What I find particularly satisfactory in this book is its adherence to the holistic code of health in mind, body, and spirit. I think we all would like to help humanity one way or another, and we are aware that there is no great point in elucidating or improving one part of the human machine and, at the same time, blinding ourselves to the fact that another vital part is meanwhile deteriorating and destroying the whole.

It has always been my feeling that no avenue should be neglected if it can lead to homeostasis, a happy equilibrium between ourselves and our surroundings, a state of steadiness and security within the limits imposed upon the human body by Nature itself.

In today's materialistic society, one must primarily convince the world that the point is not to improve our troubles with the "cost of living index"; to discover tricks through which we can get more money for less work; or to make available more of the "comforts" of civilized society, such as luxurious automobiles, television sets, or the gross national product in general. Wars will not be avoided by more sophisticated weaponry, and even disease can never be completely eradicated by improvements in pharmacology or immunotherapy or by any other purely medical means.

We must, through our collective mode, and through our devotion to human welfare, convince the great decision-makers of our times to give more attention to the quality of life. No scientific discoveries, such as nuclear fission, space travel, psychopharmacologic drugs, are in themselves good or evil for man. The great conflagrations and dangers of the future lie not in such technologic advances but in the wish or motivation of the decision-makers to use them one way or another.

I cannot think of any better way to conclude this part of my contribution and to introduce the next one than by quoting the wonderful book of John Knowles (1977) about health in the United States. In musing about why people seldom ask themselves the primordial question, "What is health?", he said:

> The term connotes bodily integrity, the absence of pain and infirmity, the state of a well-functioning and thus unremarkable organism. In a curious way, like "goodness," it can seem bland, if only because the alternative states of human affairs are so marked by drama and suffering. However bland the concept, the reality it invokes is regarded as eminently desirable. When one is in "good health" it is not even noticed; when one is not, it is desperately desired . . . .
>
> The individual has the power—indeed, the moral responsibility— to maintain his own health by the observance of simple, prudent rules of behavior relating to sleep, exercise, diet and weight, alcohol, and smoking. In addition, he should avoid where possible the long-term use of drugs. He should be aware of the dangers of stress and the need for precautionary measures during periods of sudden change, such as bereavement, divorce or new employment. He

should submit to selective medical examination and screening procedures . . . .

When all is said and done, let us not forget that he who hates sin, hates humanity. Life is meant to be enjoyed, and each one of us in the end is still able in our own country to steer his vessel to his own port of desire. But the costs of individual irresponsibility in health have now become prohibitive. The choice is individual responsibility or social failure. Responsibility and duty must gain some degree of parity with right and freedom.

3

Self-Regulation: The Response to Stress

HANS SELYE, PH.D, M.D., D.SC.

To illustrate the essence of what we have just said in Chapter 2 on "Stress—The Basis of Illness," we would like to narrate an interesting and seemingly unusual story.

Two young boys were raised by an alcoholic father. As they grew older, they moved away from that broken home, each going his own way in the world. Several years later, they happened to be interviewed separately by a psychologist who was analyzing the effects of drunkenness on children in broken homes. His research revealed that the two men were strikingly different from each other. One was a clean-living teetotaler, the other a hopeless drunk like his father. The psychologist asked each of them why he developed the way he did, and each gave an identical answer: "What else would you expect when you have had a father like mine?"

This simple story elucidates a cardinal rule implicit in stress, health, and human behavior. "It is not what happens to you in life that makes the difference. It is how you react to each circumstance you encounter that determines the result. Every human being in the same situation has the possibilities of choosing how he will react—either positively or negatively" (Schuller, 1978).

Thus, stress is not necessarily caused by stressor agents; rather, it is caused by the way stressor agents are perceived, interpreted, or appraised in each individual case (Roskies and Lazarus, N.D). Outside events and people upset some more than others, because they are looked upon and dealt with in entirely different ways. The stressors may even be the same in each case, yet the reaction will almost always be different in different people. So what is the cause of our stress—the outside agents and people, or the perception and interpretation each person brings to a given situation? If a microbe is in or around us all the time and yet causes no disease until we are exposed to stress, what is the cause of our illness—the microbe or the stress? These are the questions we must ask ourselves today.

We have spent many years of research, some of them very fruitful years, studying the so-called causes of stress, and it has turned out that we have all along been investigating its physiologic or organic mechanisms and manifestations. However, it is by no means implied that we should terminate our studies of stress mechanisms and manifestations to concentrate on other possibly more meaningful and rewarding areas.

The point being made here is that we have clarified many, if not most, of the stress mechanisms in physiology and, particularly, in endocrinology, but these perspectives are necessarily narrow. "Each time there occurred a rapid spurt in the understanding of some of these forces, microbes for instance, the focus shifted from the interacting whole to functions of the parts. During the last century, the rapid development of methodology and sophistication in approaches to individual parts and isolated mechanisms drowned the earlier concepts that saw the balance of health and disease at the organismal level and as the result of man's interaction with the myriad forces in his environment" (Wolf and Goodell, 1976).

An essentially holistic approach would therefore be at the

very basis of our understanding of the causes and mechanisms of stress. The present biomedical model is being increasingly attacked as being too reductionistic and, indeed, too simplistic (Engel, 1977). Interestingly enough, many of those who question the biomedical model cannot be brushed aside as inconsequential, anti-establishment types, for they come from within the very ranks of the biomedical system. This crisis in medicine stems mainly from the large-scale exclusion of all variables other than the somatic as being the cause(s) of disease. Such an approach is evidently inadequate for society's health and well-being, because it assumes that biomedical interventions are specifically directed to the cause(s) of disease. Furthermore, its main thrust is cure rather than prevention, but, above all, it fails to answer a question of great import to the stress researcher: What is the actual cause of stress?

THE CAUSES OF STRESS

Biomedical Research

As the so-called father of the stress concept, I have often been asked this question: What are the causes of stress?

Our stress research originated in the 1930s. In these four intervening decades, we have found answers to many perplexing questions. We have established the physiologic triad of stress in experimental animals, and we have analyzed its pathways and mechanisms with a living organism, the rat. This careful dissection of stress has given us many experimental models of striking similarity to the stress disorders of man. The significance of these advances is perhaps taken for granted, much like the prescription of corticoid preparations and the common use of certain biomedical antistress interventions.

In any event, we have succeeded in determining many of the basic physiologic pathways of stress. We have been able to prove the significant roles played by the pituitary, the adrenals, and other endocrine glands during the stress reaction (Selye, 1976; 1956). We have elucidated the basic functions of certain stress hormones, and now, with the rapid acceleration of stress research by other institutes all over the world, many new biochemical pathways have been uncovered. The most diverse physiologic and psychogenic stressors are now being studied, some in their natural form, others under specially created conditions, and their nonspecific effects are being carefully monitored in relation to innumerable physicochemical parameters. Furthermore, the list of chemical, morphologic, and functional manifestations of stress has grown to such unmanageable proportions that it is becoming increasingly difficult to wade through the stress literature just to get an overview of the entire field.

Stress research has met with great success in a vast number of areas, particularly in explaining the nervous and hormonal mechanisms or pathways of stress. I take great pride in some of my former students who have distinguished themselves in stress research. Some of them have easily forged ahead of their old teacher. I refer especially to the work of Roger Guillemin in elucidating the structure of the endorphins, which some believe may be the first mediators of stress. To some extent, they could be early mediators, but essentially they represent a physicochemical mechanism; they are not the cause of stress, because they are themselves triggered by an elusive first mediator and, hence, are part of the organism's response to stress (Rossier, Bloom, and Guillemin, ND). We have come no closer to it than that.

We have yet to discover the entire neuroendocrine process, and then we will have to ascertain how these neuroendocrinologic mechanisms and behavior are intricately related to perception, appraisal, and interpretation (Roskies and Lazarus, ND). We need to travel beyond the mechanisms of disturbed visceral function. We must discover why and how certain symbolically significant life experiences unleash the forces of stress and stress hormones.

Our own investigations have meanwhile shed no light on the identity of the first mediator. We believe the answer lies partially in the realm of the biomedical model. Finding the answer would need cooperation from the other branches of medicine, notably, neuroendocrinology, psychology, and the other behavioral sciences.

We have witnessed a staggering growth of these disciplines and have reported some of the key findings in a recent encyclopedia of stress (Selye, 1976). This volume was written with the belief that the specialized areas of stress research need not be exclusive of one another. Some active form of cooperation and a major exchange of knowledge seemed to be required. In this volume, the reader will find an adequate overview of the biomedical model, one that is impressive in its breadth and scope, yet flexible enough to permit cooperation between these disciplines.

Not satisfied with this one effort to bring together all the disciplines under one roof, we proceeded to create the International Institute of Stress as a central data bank for all the stress literature in existence. Above all, the purpose of the Institute is to build a coordination center for all of stress research, a center that would pool all the information on stress and what causes it. The great and urgent need for multidisciplinary teamwork is recognized as the imperative for a new type of medicine.

At this point in time, there are many such specialists keenly motivated in a joint, holistic approach, so that the human resources are not lacking. I would derive considerable joy and eustress if, through this cooperation, we could eventually find out just what causes stress. It is my hope that we will soon make out the true identity of the "first mediator."

Meanwhile, we can pride ourselves that our team has started to make some basic contributions to the biomedical model. Our stress research has taught us at least three most obvious lessons:

1. That our bodies can meet the most diverse aggressions with the same adaptive defense mechanisms.
2. That we can dissect these mechanisms so as to identify their ingredient parts in objectively measurable physical and chemical terms, such as

changes in the structure of organs or in the production of certain hormones.

3. That we need this kind of information to lay the scientific foundations for a new type of medicine, whose essence is to combat suffering and disease by strengthening the body's own defenses against stress.

Once we have learned that, in a given situation, an excess of a certain hormone is needed to maintain health, we can inject that hormone whenever the body is unable to manufacture enough of it. Conversely, once we have recognized that a disease is due to the exaggerated adaptive activity in some hormone-producing gland, we can remove the offending organ or try to block its activity by drugs or other measures.

In terms of human behavior, this would amount to much the same thing as strengthening the mind, the psyche, so as not to depend upon outside interventions. It is said that ours is a "left brain society," a label that emphasizes the scientific model: structure, discipline, study of detail, careful appraisal of facts, observation, and reporting of what we see. Perhaps the emphasis on left brain activity has resulted in the atrophy of man's right brain, causing a disharmony or imbalance. We need right brain activity as much as we do left brain activity, for we need our intuitive flashes, our creative impulses, after subconscious digestion of left brain input. All great scientific discoveries start as the intuitive product of right brain activity (Selye, 1975).

Einstein and others have said that what we observe is partly the result of what the observer's participation is in the observation. Thus, we are constantly involved in left brain activity to the neglect of the right brain. Perhaps we need to develop right brain activity so that both sides get into balance, each performing its function as needed.

On the physiologic level at least, we now know that the body possesses a complex machinery of self-regulating checks and balances. These are remarkably effective in adjusting ourselves to virtually anything that can happen to us in life. But often this machinery does not work perfectly: Sometimes our responses are too weak, so that they do not offer adequate protection; at other times, they are too strong, so that we actually hurt ourselves by our own excessive reactions to stress.

We first have to know how a machine works in order to adjust or repair it. This is, of course, also true of the stress machinery with which man combats the wear and tear of whatever he does in this world. Therefore, the most obvious, tangible outcome of our work was to show that stress can be dissected into its elements, and that the knowledge derived from this analysis helps us to speed up a part which lags behind or to restrain another which goes too far. But therapy with hormones and drugs or the surgical removal of endocrine glands are certainly not procedures that the individual could prescribe for himself (Selye, 1956).

Many books and courses are now available that could offer valuable help and direction to anyone interested in starting a stress-reduction program (Brown, 1977; Truch, 1977; Oates, 1976; Luthe, 1977). To say that the individual should follow any one of these measures would be tantamount to admitting that a given stress meter or test could monitor all the stress reactions in body and mind. There is no such simple solution, no ready-made success formula that would suit one and all. Not yet anyway. But it would help to know that a great deal of today's stress is self-inflicted and therefore avoidable.

ANTI-STRESS INTERVENTIONS

To a large extent, the damage caused by the excessive stress of disease can only be combatted by the physician. We do have tranquilizers that can reduce anxiety and tension, and we know of a variety of specific drugs that can combat stress-induced high blood pressure, peptic ulcers, mental diseases, headaches, and many other disturbances usually caused by stress in predisposed individuals. But all of these so-called wonder drugs are of limited efficacy and have some undesirable side effects. In particular, they are not directed *per se* at the causes of stress. They are generally interventions after the fact has occurred, after disease has set in.

Countless stress tests and questionnaires have been developed in order to help people appraise their stress situations. (In our Documentation Service, we have articles describing some 500 of them!) There are also various complex instruments, known as stress meters or stress polygraphs, but they can register only a few indicators that are usually, though not always, characteristic of stress. Of course, the more signs and symptoms are measured, the more reliable the general picture becomes. But all these tests fail to indicate the very significant fact that it is our *ability to cope* with the demands made by the events in our lives, not their quality and the intensity of the resulting measurable physiologic changes, that counts. What matters is not so much what happens to us, but how we perceive it!

According to experience, the stress of our lives can be self-perceived as:

1. General irritability, hyperexcitation, or depression.
2. Pounding of the heart, an indicator of high blood pressure (often due to stress).
3. Dryness of the throat and mouth.
4. Impulsive behavior, aggressiveness, emotional instability. (Emotion wins over logic.)
5. The overpowering urge to cry or to run and hide.
6. Inability to concentrate, flight of thoughts, and general disorientation.
7. Accident proneness. Under great stress (eustress or distress), we are more likely to have accidents at work or while driving a car. This is also a very important reason why pilots and air traffic controllers must be carefully checked for their stress status.
8. Feelings of unreality, weakness, or dizziness.
9. Fatigue and loss of "joie de vivre."
10. "Floating anxiety"; that is to say, we are afraid, although we do not know exactly what we are afraid of.
11. Emotional tension and alertness, a feeling of being "keyed up."

12. Sexual difficulties, amenorrhea, impotence, premenstrual tension, the "Casanova" complex, nymphomania.*

13. Trembling; nervous ticks.

14. Tendency to be easily startled by small sounds.

15. High-pitched, nervous laughter.

16. Stuttering and other speech difficulties, which are frequently stress-induced.

17. Bruxism or grinding of the teeth.

18. Insomnia, which is usually a consequence of being "keyed up."

19. Hypermotility, or hyperkinesia, an increased tendency to move about or gesticulate without any apparent reason.

20. Excessive sweating.

21. The frequent need to urinate.

22. Diarrhea, constipation, indigestion, queasiness in the stomach, and sometimes even vomiting. All are signs of disturbed gastrointestinal function, which eventually may lead to such severe diseases of adaptation as peptic ulcers, ulcerative colitis, and so on.

23. Loss of or excessive appetite, which shows itself soon in alterations of body weight—either excessive leanness or obesity. Some people lose their appetite during stress because of gastrointestinal malfunction, whereas others eat excessively as a kind of diversion, to deviate their attention from the stressor situation. Besides, a well-filled stomach and intestine shift a great deal of blood to the abdomen, resulting in a relative decrease in brain circulation, which tranquilizes by decreasing mental alertness.

24. Pain in the neck or lower back. In conversational English, the expressions, "This business is an awful headache" or "He gives me a pain in the neck" are not merely colorful verbalizations but are based on actual experience. For example, pain in the neck or back is usually due to increases in muscular tension that can be objectively measured by the physician with the electromyogram (EMG).

25. Migraine headaches.

26. Increased smoking.*

*Compiled mainly from *The Stress of Life* (see References for Chapter 3) up-dated by the Library and Documentation Service of the International Institute of Stress. Further information available upon request from the Institute.

27. Increased use of various prescribed medications, such as tranquilizers or amphetamines.

28. Alcohol or drug addiction. Like the phenomenon of overeating, increased and excessive alcohol consumption or the use of various psychotropic drugs is a common manifestation of exposure to stressors beyond our natural endurance. Here again, we are actually dealing with "flight" reactions, known as diversion or deviation, to which we resort presumably because they help us to forget the cause of our distress and tend to temporarily replace it by the eustress of psychic elation or at least tranquilization.

29. Nightmares.

30. Neurotic behavior or even severe mental illness (Selye, 1956).

There are four basic aspects of the stress of life, although in their most characteristic nonspecific nature, they all depend upon the same central phenomenon (Selye, 1977). This might be illustrated in a simple diagram, as shown in Figure 3–1. A number of signs of stress, particularly of the more dangerous distress, can serve to monitor our condition throughout life. Depending upon our "conditioning," we all respond differently to general demands. But on the whole, each of us tends to respond particularly with one set of signs, caused by the malfunction of whatever happens to be the most vulnerable part in our machinery, and when those signs appear, it is time to heed the body's warning.

Figure 3.1 The four basic aspects of stress.

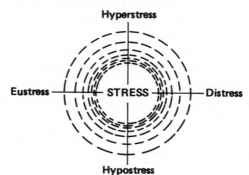

Everyone must learn to recognize what for him or her is "overstress" (hyperstress)—when he or she has exceeded the limits of his or her adaptability—or "understress" (hypostress)—when he or she suffers from lack of self-realization (physical immobility, boredom, sensory deprivation). Being overwrought is just as bad as being frustrated by the inability to express oneself and find free outlets for one's innate muscular or mental energy (Selye, 1977).

Still, the individual's coping processes may fail him, and then he is forced to seek help from the biomedical model. He is given invaluable assistance, but hospitalized medicine can never become the mainstay of society's health. No institution can ever hope to assume such a responsibility, for it remains a very personal matter between the individual and his environment. The ultimate custodian of society's health, then, is the individual, the effort he puts into being a healthy participant in a certain life process.

Must we become alarmed if we see a breakdown of health at the individual's stress level? I believe the time has come to be concerned about our future and its quality. We should not assume that it is natural for a patient to give up his health responsibilities entirely to organized medical institutions.

As I said in *The Stress of Life* (1956), "adaptability (what some prefer to call "coping") is probably the most distinctive characteristic of life. In maintaining the independence and individuality of natural units, none of the great forces of inanimate matter are as successful as that alertness and adaptability to change which we designate as life—and the loss of which is death. Indeed, there is perhaps even a certain parallelism between the degree of aliveness and the extent of adaptability in every animal—in every man."

The individual can largely control his physical and mental reactions by acquiring a more philosophical, healthier attitude toward the pressures and urgencies of everyday life. The initiative must, of course, come from the individual himself. He must be willing to reorganize his daily priorities, he must be willing to slow down or accelerate his pace of life, and he must even be willing to accept a complete change of lifestyle. If these "demands" for adaptation and survival cannot be met, humanity can never have any hope for a better future. We would not need ingenious nuclear devices to eliminate the human race—oblivion would come just as surely and swiftly if we allowed stress to proliferate and devour our well-being.

> The Western World . . . is in the throes of a social upheaval of unparalleled proportions. Julian Huxley has pointed out that the tempo of human evolution and the rate of change in human affairs are ever accelerating, and Sir George Thomson, the British physicist and Nobel laureate, has compared the impact of current changes on human life to the invention of agriculture in the Neolithic age. Standards of behavior, of individual freedom, of the degree of acceptance of authority, of the experiences of the senses and of the very patterns of living are now undergoing the most profound alterations. Since the rate of change of events, of attitudes and of standards is so much more rapid than has ever occurred previously, the impact of these upheavals on society as a whole and on any specific individual is more profound than that experienced during earlier historical movements, which evolved over decades or centuries" (Braunwald, 1972).

Physical and Emotional Stressors

The more immediate everyday stressors could be divided into two major categories: physical and emotional stressors. The former include "noxious" agents, such as trauma; poisons; near-poisons (caffeine, alcohol, nicotine, and other social drugs): hormones and hormone-like substances; dietary factors; physical elements, including extremes of temperature, ultraviolet and infrared radiation from sunlight, nuclear radiation, x-rays, pollution, hypoxia, decreased barometric pressure, hyperbaric oxygenation, electricity, electroshock, noise, magnetism, airblasts, vibration, compression, decompression, gravity, circadian variations, seasonal variations, meteorologic influences, burns, viruses, bacteria, muscular exertion, restraint, captivity, crowding, isolation, relocation and travel, urbanization, occupations (air traffic control, shift work, unemployment, retirement), driving, accidents, catastrophes, sex, pregnancy and lactation, age, genetics, race, constitution, and many more.

Some of these physical stressors overlap to a large extent with neuropsychologic stimuli, such as pain, grief, anxiety, anticipation, fear, hate, anger, boredom, sleep deprivation, sensory deprivation, pleasure, worry about social taboos, and so on (Selye, 1976).

It would be virtually impossible to arrive at a sharp demarcation between these two broad categories. Although some of the physical stressors have few directly noxious effects, the changes they elicit alter basic and established relations between man and his environment. Thus, the stressors are potentially noxious; they engender stress and often evoke major defense reactions inappropriate in kind and amount to the type of behavior one might expect.

> The stress accruing from a situation is based . . . on the way the affected subject perceives it; perception depends upon a multiplicity of factors, including the genetic equipment, basic individual needs and longings, earlier conditioning influences, and a host of life experiences and cultural pressures. No one of these can be singled out for exclusive emphasis. The common denominator of "stress disorders" is reaction to circumstances of threatening significance to the organism.

> The particular adaptative pattern evoked by a noxious agent or threat is the result of past life experience which conditions individuals to react in specific ways. Hence, "etiology" in disease becomes a function not merely of precipitating incident and setting, but largely of the past of the individual and his stock (Wolf and Goodell, 1968).

Precipitating incidents always have the potential of being stressors. A person' reaction to those incidents determines whether there is stress.

> We should not consider stress as *imposed* upon the organism, but as its *response* to internal or external processes which reach those threshold levels that strain its physiological integrative capacities close to or beyond their limits (Basowitz et al., 1955).

Meeting a challenge may result in a gain or loss, depending upon our reactions, and it is largely within our power to respond constructively once we know the rules of the game. On the automatic, involuntary level, the gain is accomplished through chemical responses (immunity, destruction of poisons, healing of wounds, etc.), which ensure survival and minimal tissue damage under a given set of circumstances. These reactions are either spontaneous or they must be guided by an experienced specialist. But it is even possible that we could train ourselves to react in a positive and creative manner at certain stressful periods by merely willing ourselves to do so.

The ancient Greek philosophers clearly recognized that the most important but perhaps also the most difficult thing was "to know thyself." Only he who knows himself can profit by the advice of Matthew Arnold: "Resolve to be thyself and know that he who finds himself, loses his misery." After all, "it is in the mind that we confront a problem, not in the stomach or the joints—though the mind may call on the stomach for a solution, or may pass the problem on to the joints if a solution fails" (McQuade and Aikman, 1974).

Psychoanalysis has demonstrated, perhaps better than any other branch of medicine, that *knowing what hurts you has a curative value in itself.* The psychoanalyst helps you to understand how previous experiences—which may have led to subconscious conflicts, sometimes very early in childhood—can continue almost indefinitely to cause mental or even physical disease. But once you realize the mechanism of your mental conflicts, they cease to bother you.

Sigmund Freud's efforts to develop a branch of medicine on the basis of this concept provided the first major focus on the effects of past experiences as well as physical symptomatology upon human behavior. He gave us a model which is less useful now as a clinical procedure, but then it served to highlight the influence of thought and emotion on our health and well-being. Of course, here we are dealing with diseases of adaptation. Our failure to adjust ourselves correctly to life situations is at the very root of the disease-producing conflicts. Psychoanalysis cures because it helps us to adapt ourselves to what has happened.

All this is sufficiently well known, at least in regard to mental reactions, and deserves no further comment. But "to know thyself" includes the body. Most people fail to realize that "to know thy body" also has an inherent curative value. Take a familiar example. Many people have joints that tend to crack at almost every movement. By concentrating on this unexplained condition, a person can worry himself into believing that he has a crippling arthritis. If, on the other hand, some understanding physician explains to him that his cracking sensations have no tendency to become worse, the disease is practically cured—just by the knowledge of its trifling nature (Selye, 1956).

At some time or other, almost everybody has had some insignificant allergic condition of the skin, cardiac palpitations, or intestinal upsets. Any of these conditions can cause serious illness through somatopsychic reactions, merely because not knowing what is wrong makes us anxious. Every physician knows from experience how much can be done for a patient by just taking time to explain the mechanism of his symptoms, which thereby lose the frightening element of mystery.

Today, many people abuse drugs, and unless a physician prescribes some kind of pill or surgical intervention, he loses his patient's trust. Yet medicine and surgery are not the only means available to maintain the well-being of humanity. The great majority of diseases for which patients seek medical help are, at least in part, psychosomatic. If someone suffers from a peptic ulcer, for example, it is not only the ulcer that should be cured but also the patient's reaction to the life events that caused his susceptibility to this particular stress-induced disease. Here, the ulcer is a symptom, not a cause of the disease.

It is possible to relieve psychosomatically induced peptic ulcers, high blood pressure, migraine headaches, asthma attacks, mental disturbances, and many other diseases merely by using drugs or surgical interventions. However, to use only these methods would be wrong, just as wrong as treating "the fevers" with antipyretics: These will reduce the fever but will not cure the typhoid or tuberculosis that has provoked it.

With most psychosomatic diseases, it is the philosophy of life, the code of behavior of the patient, that is really at fault.

Living beings are motivated by a variety of impulses, among which the selfish desire to maintain oneself, to stay alive and happy, is one of the most important. The satisfaction of our instinctive drives, the need for self-expression, the impulse to collect wealth and acquire power, the need to do some constructive work, the desire to fulfill whatever we consider our purpose, and many other motives are conjointly responsible for our actions. It is therefore healthy to take stock of these desires and to analyze their justification and biologic value in maintaining our homeostasis—our equilibrium—within ourselves and within society.

With the ease of communications today, we are constantly bombarded by new methods of "coping with life." Sociologists, psychologists, and journalists tell us that, as the population grows and the pace of life quickens, the world is becoming an increasingly frustrating place. Whether or not this is because our troubles as a whole are greater now than in the past, we would certainly all like to rid our lives of the bad effects of stress and enjoy as much eu-stress as possible.

To meet this longing, new techniques spring up daily, all claiming to reduce stress. Among these, some are worth taking seriously, others are nothing but fads. Most of these methods teach us—some more effectively than others—how to deal with "the cruel world." However, our goal should not be merely to master techniques for shutting out reality but to devise a better lifestyle that can change reality.

Some people find sufficient diversion in leisure activities to keep their own stress level to a desirable point. But many of us have an irresistible drive to seek stress in the form of challenge, competition, and the like, even when we are supposed to be playing. It is a common experience for a person under pressure to get the feeling of merely wasting time when indulging in leisure activities. Not everyone knows how to play or how to enjoy the passive experiences of music, spectator sports, or reading. When the pent-up energy has no outlet, these are the people who turn to drugs, violence, and other destructive activities. But there are alternatives: some good, some not so good.

Smoking, alcohol, tranquilizers, and eating all help to relieve distress in those who suffer from nervous excitation. The trouble here is that these remedies tend to become problems themselves through their habit-forming properties.

In recent years, some of the Eastern methods of stress reduction have become very popular. Ironically, these ancient methods of relieving stress and promoting tranquility are finding their way into many laboratories and clinics. Innumerable scientific investigations are now claiming that transcendental meditation (TM), yoga, and other self-regulating techniques do have a wide range of beneficial effects on those who practice them. We do not believe that these methods can cure disease, but they certainly could help the individual to obtain some relief from excessive stress by controlling such basic functions as breathing, heart rate, blood pressure, and the electrical activity of the brain.

If we can indeed learn to control the vital functions of our bodies, then we have moved a great step closer to the prevention of disease. Autohypnosis, breathing exercises, autogenic training, and biofeedback can certainly help us to strengthen our defenses against stress. They cannot totally eliminate distress because challenge and tension are a part of life. But by mobilizing energy as a positive force, we can use the wisdom of the body to prevent disease (Cannon, 1939).

Everybody will arrive at this aim in a somewhat different manner, one characteristic of his own individuality. Some come to understand their inner needs through meditation and silence; others may only find their own stress level through danger signs such as insomnia, irritability, indigestion, headaches, or depression. Judging what is best for us personally is a matter of training through experience.

A Mind-Over-Body Approach

It is quite clear by now that stress is a matter of perception and, that being the case, that the body can be instructed to react at a proper level by educating the mind. It is becoming increasingly evident that the human body is pliable, changeable, and capable of being altered through mental conditioning. Experts in various fields are now exploring the possibility of curing disease by mind-over-body treatment.

Even physical fitness in all its various forms works on the premise that the muscles (and internal organs) can be strengthened, toned up, and manipulated to an attractive shape. If we can accept this principle in terms of the body, it should be relatively easy to train and shape the mind, to loosen its inhibitions and limitations and to gear up the mental faculties to cope with any and every demand. To be physically fit evidently requires a certain amount of mental organization. There can be no question that the muscular system is under the direct control of the nervous system. By changing our consciousness, by altering our awareness, we will have changed our perception of the "hard realities of life." An altered state of consciousness or awareness could well be the result of balanced left and right brain activities, giving us a properly balanced view of life.

It is important, indeed it is vital, to learn how to handle our emotional tensions—to know and to accept our physical and emotional limitations. All this is easier said than done. But understanding is the first step. As we reach a better understanding of the common emotional and physical stresses and are able to recognize them instead of trying to ignore them, we shall begin to see a reduction of those illnesses that strike out at us through our own inner conflicts. We can all, in our own way, practice an important bit of preventive medicine by applying this knowledge to ourselves (Selye, 1977).

When we have exceeded our stress level, it is not easy to tune down or up. Everybody is familiar with the feeling of being keyed up from nervous tension. This process is comparable to raising the key of a violin by tightening the strings. We say that our muscles limber up during exercise and that we are thrilled by great emotional experiences. All this prepares us for better peak accomplishments.

On the other hand, there is the tingling sensation, the jitteriness, when we are keyed up too much. This impairs our work and even prevents us from getting a rest. Just what happens to us when we are tense?

Being keyed up is a very real sensation which must have a physicochemical basis. It has not yet been fully analyzed. but we know that at times of tension our adrenals produce an excess of both catecholamines (e.g., adrenalin) and corticoids. We also know that taking either adrenalin or corticoids can reproduce a very similar sensation of being keyed up and excitable.

Thus, a person who is given large doses of cortisone for some allergic or rheumatoid condition often finds it difficult to sleep. He may even become abnormally euphoric; that is, carried away by an unreasonable sense of well-being and buoyancy, which interferes with sleep and is not unlike that caused by being very slightly drunk. Later, somnolence and a sense of deep depression may follow.

We know now that identifiable chemical compounds—the hormones produced during the acute alarm reaction phase of the G.A.S.—possess this property of first keying up the system for action and then causing a depression. Both these effects may be of great practical value to the body: It is necessary to be keyed up for peak accomplishments, but it is equally important to be keyed down by the secondary phase of depression, which prevents us from carrying on too long at top speed.

The known hormones are probably not the only regulators of our emotional level. Besides, we do not yet know enough about their workings to justify any attempt at regulating our emotional key by taking hormones. Still, it is instructive to realize that stress stimulates our glands to make hormones, which can induce a kind of drunkenness. The fact is that a person can be intoxicated by his own stress hormones, and this sort of drunkenness has caused much more harm to society than that induced by alcohol or other social stimulants.

We are on our guard against external toxicants, but hormones are parts of our bodies. It takes wisdom to recognize and overcome the foe which fights from within. Intoxication by stress is sometimes unavoidable and usually insidious. We can quit alcohol, and, even if we do take some, at least we can count the glasses; but is impossible to avoid stress as long as we are alive (Selye, 1956).

The Wisdom of the Body

It could hardly be mere coincidence that in his epilogue to *The Wisdom of the Body* (1939), Walter Cannon expressed his conviction that the behavior and philosophy of man could and should be guided to a large extent by the living organism. "Might it not be useful," he asked, "to examine other forms of organization—industrial, domestic or social—in the light of the organization of the body?" After reviewing various philosophical and political systems designed to maintain the homeostasis necessary for the happiness of mankind, he concluded that "the multiplicity of these schemes is itself proof that no satisfactory single scheme has been suggested by anybody."

I certainly agree with Cannon that the greatest advantage of developing specialized organs in complex living beings, including man, is that each part can better concentrate on its own special activity (locomotion, digestion, excretion of waste products) if it is supplied, through the blood stream, with the general necessities of life (oxygen, energy-yielding nutrients). However, this advantage becomes possible only if other systems coordinate all specialized activities through nervous impulses harmonized by the feedback mechanisms of the central nervous system that show where there is an excess or an unsatisfied demand.

It is this great capacity for adaptation (or coping) that makes life possible on all levels of complexity. It is the basis of homeostasis and of resistance to stress. This is probably why, in the course of evolution, colonies of individual cells got together to form a single cooperative community in which competition was amply overcompensated by mutual assistance, because each member of the group could depend upon the others for help. Different cells specialized, each to undertake different functions: some to look after food intake and digestion; others to provide the means for respiration, locomotion, and defense; still others to coordinate the activities of the entire colony. Among the individual cells of such closely knit complex bodies, egoism and altruism became, virtually synonymous. There can be no motive for competitive struggles among cells that depend upon one another and share everything, even a single life. In fact, the evolution of diverse species was largely dependent upon the development of processes that permitted many cells to live in harmony, in balance, with a minimum of stress between them, serving their own best interests by ensuring the survival of the entire complex structure.

At the same time, there developed an interdependence (symbiosis, mutualism) between two or more individuals of completely different species. This form of mutually useful *altruistic egoism* is extremely widespread in Nature. One could enumerate countless examples of it, but a few will suffice. There are instances of symbiosis between various microorganisms as well as between bacteria and higher animals. The normal bacteria that live in the intestine of a mammal not only reduce ingested plants and animals to a form usable by the host, but they also provide their host with an immunity to disease-producing bacteria that is lacking in animals kept artificially in a germ-free atmosphere.

One could mention many similar associations among all sorts of species along the evolutionary scale. As for the individuals within a single species, the life of bees, ants, termites, and other social animals could never have reached its present stage of sophisticated development without division of labor and collaboration.

However, from our point of view, the most interesting interdependence that has developed in the course of evolution is that among human beings. Each of us has his or her own ambitions and requirements, which often clash and become the major source of interpersonal stress. Naturally, the best solution to this problem would be perfect teamwork and mutual understanding, but, despite all the codes of conduct offered by various religions, philosophies, and political systems, interpersonal relations remain very unsatisfactory. The stress of living with one another still represents one of the greatest causes of dis-tress (Selye, 1974).

The indispensability of disciplined, orderly, mutual cooperation is best illustrated by its opposite—the development of a cancerous growth, whose most characteristic feature is that it cares only for itself. Hence, it feeds on the other parts of its own host until it kills the host and thus commits biologic suicide, since a cancer cell cannot live except within the body in which it started its reckless, egoistic development (Selye, 1974). The same is true of many bacteria and viruses.

The evolution of sophisticated systems of mutual aid between the parts of a single organism minimized internal stress; that is, it diminished the demands made on the body for the avoidance of internal frictions so as to permit a harmonious coexistence of all parts of the unit (Selye, 1974). I believe that similar principles govern cooperation between entire nations: Just as a person's health depends upon the harmonious conduct of the organs within his body, so must the relations between individual people—and, by extension, between the members of families, tribes, and nations—be harmonized by self-integrity, peaceful cooperation, and balance, leading to "altruistic egoism," which automatically removes all motives and impulses for revolutions and wars.

Viewed from the pinnacle of the eternal general laws governing Nature, we are all suprisingly alike. Nature is the fountainhead of all our problems and solutions. The closer we keep to her, the better we realize that, despite the apparently enormous divergencies in interpretation and explanation, her laws have always prevailed and can never become obsolete. Consequently, I feel that the rules we must follow have to be based on the laws of Nature. We are part of Nature and therefore cannot disregard her laws with impunity.

THE MASTERY OF STRESS

A Holistic Prescription

Because of his highly developed central nervous system, man can consciously direct his actions according to the laws of Nature. He also possesses the natural forces of cooperation based on his biologic structure and function. He has the natural ability to be in perfect harmony and balance with himself, with his ecology. Indeed, this is a natural state of all life forces.

The present state of human affairs has come about because of interferences in our belief systems. We have been taught for too long to live along the lines of survival of the fittest, of competition for the top spot. We therefore cannot love our neighbors if we perceive them as threats. Our belief systems have been altered away from our natural state. We must now learn to regain that natural state by consciousness expansion: We must recognize just who we are, and we must know that we are capable of positive thought and action, that we can generate good feelings towards ourselves and others, in order to get back to the harmonious existence of a life force. Once we have evolved to such a new, healthy state of perception and awareness, creating a new image of peace within ourselves and all around us, we will find ourselves following the natural principles of altruistic egoism. This is a natural consequence of a heightened state of awareness of oneself, of better harmony and balance, which creates peace and love and all the other attributes we sorely miss and are desperately looking for.

We have been so overwhelmed with the abnormalities of modern day living that we have come to believe that the abnormal is the norm. We overlook the fact that natural harmony, balance, and homeostasis are the norm. The abnormalities created by our negative thought processes produce the chaos in our lives. That is why the trend today is towards Eastern philosophies, where people seek to develop right brain activity, the intuitive side of themselves, and to seek answers in areas other than structure, function, and scientific discipline, so as to achieve that balance. The capacity is already within us. We only need to remove the debris of distorted thought processes we have collected over the years.

We must realign our belief systems to perceive agents as not being necessarily stressful. We will then be able to respond in an appropriate manner to whatever stressful situations life may have in store for us. We will easily recognize exactly what is causing our distress and we will act accordingly. The conversion of our perceptual capabilities will change dis-tress into eu-stress, a positive life force vital to man.

We cannot continue to confine ourselves to molecular approaches and treatments. We must give free rein to the reinforcing medicine practiced by those who work with belief systems, for these are just as important as the biomedical practices. Perhaps we even need "holistic doctors of health" to treat our disoriented belief systems, which all too often make us do strange, "unnatural" things because we are fearful or insecure. We need to develop "a new generation of physicians capable of a broad understanding of human ecology, as well as of highly refined specialized skills, capable of being lifetime students of the progress of medical science, and capable of coordinating with a host of paramedical agencies an effective health program for individuals" (Wolf and Goodell, 1976). These specialists will be capable of molding our belief system by showing us that our physical work and our realities are essentially thought processes or rationalizations. They will demonstrate that our conscious self-protecting measures sometimes produce distorted, dislocated views which must be removed so that the natural life forces may work in balance.

By believing in the need for balance, we can change our responses, and then people around us can no longer react to us in the old way. They will have to change, since we will not be responding in the usual, expected manner. We can get our realities to change by first changing ourselves, by expanding our awareness and our consciousness for productive thoughts, ideas, and aspirations. This would explain why most stress-reduction programs enable the individual to use his logical faculties "to prevent the stress reaction from escalating beyond a practical minimum level in any situation, and to acquire new neurological skills which more or less regulate the body's activation level at will" (Albrecht, 1979).

Biofeedback, autogenic therapy, TM, autohypnosis, and so on can serve as additional training aids to relieve stress. In other words, they would have the effect of isolating stress and reducing or converting it.

If all these personal or individual health measures do not succeed, then we must fall back on the biomedical model, seeking the aid of those who understand disease processes, pharmacology, and the clinical aspects of pain and suffering. Thus, we must look at health from all three levels:

1. As belief systems.
2. As voluntary preventive measures.
3. As medical interventions.

We should certainly explore all three levels to their fullest extent.

Those who perceive this world as cruel, anxious, tense, or threatening need to alter their basic beliefs. Otherwise they create an environment of cruelty, anxiety, tension, and threats, attracting people around them who are in the same consciousness. Changes in belief systems would have long-lasting effects, as compared to the temporary interventions of the biomedical model. Still, both approaches would reinforce one another's strengths. Such a cooperation would teach people how they could help themselves rather than teaching them how to place their dependence entirely upon socialized medicine, drugs, surgery, and so forth. The individual would have a clear, more intuitive behavioral direction. His misguided perceptions would be removed, strengthening his defenses against stress and allowing him to assume more control over his condition in life, his port of destination. His behavior would be directed by positive internal regulation.

Such self-regulation, this awareness of internal processes, will reduce the likelihood of diseases of adaptation. It will get people back on their feet again, back to better health, able to see a more peaceful quality in the nature of their fellowmen. The achievement of a better harmony and balance in world affairs will not come from governments. It is going to come from each one's own personal consciousness, growing and expanding to a higher state of being.

The success of a good life is based on validation by the self. If the center is fulfilled, the outer spaces of our lives rest in tranquility. In self-regulation, then, lies the most promising answer to mankind's health and happiness. It is a grave responsibility worthy of that noble race we call man.

In conclusion, I would like to quote Harold G. Wolff (1960), whose work should be a great inspiration to us in coping with the stress of our lives. He said:

> The unifying concept about man in relation to his environment . . . is grounded on the recognition of the purposive, goal-directed activity inherent in living things, from the unfolding of a seed to man's pursuit of his highest aspirations. It is a concept in keeping with the facts of the goal-directed and self-regulating organization of all biologic systems, recognizing on the one hand the forces within the system that direct its development, form and functions, and on the other hand the molding influence of outside forces and changing relationships. It is a concept that requires that man be sensitive to the unfolding of his individual patterns, the kind of person he is, and the direction in which he can move. In a narrower sense, such a concept illuminates the nature of disease and gives it meaning; in a broader sense, it can serve as a basis for a philosophy. It is a concept that accounts for the destructive, inappropriate use of adaptive patterns when the individual perceives himself as threatened, not only where his own ends or self-survival are in question, but as well when spiritual or moral values are jeopardized. Sickness may ensue and his life may be dramatically shortened in his struggles for issues beyond himself. His aspirations and appetite for adventure may engender ominous conflict yet make possible growth to undefined limits.

The recognition of the role of stress and its all pervasive influence in the etiology of disease and illness has resulted in more attention devoted to self-regulatory mechanisms.

The fact that people can regulate many of their body functions, until recently thought to be beyond such conscious control, is of enormous significance to health care. It may herald a new age in medical care, a refocus of attention to the person instead of to the condition. With the growing importance of biofeedback and other self-direction methods, new opportunities are presented for patients to participate in their own recovery from illness, and in their own well-being. It also provides an excellent means of encouraging an individual to assume more responsibility for his or her health, not by lecture or admonition but by demonstration of the control he or she possesses through experiencing it.

The scientific research establishing the value of these approaches should have a marked influence in assisting the physician with alternative treatment possibilities that will augment the traditional modes.

Dr. Stroebel highlights what some of these self-regulation methods are, as well as their appropriate use in helping people to help themselves.

4

Voluntary Self-Regulation of Stress

CHARLES F. STROEBEL, PH.D., M.D.

"Stress" has been described by Hans Selye (Selye, 1974) as a precipitating or potentiating factor in the onset and expression of many forms of illness. Indeed, an estimated fifty to seventy percent of all complaints in general medical practice are stress-related, so that the symptom might not have occurred, or would have been less severe, had the stress not been present. Unfortunately, most of us have come to accept such stress as an unavoidable consequence of the pace and complexity of Western life. Need this be inevitable? The practical alternatives in this chapter lead to one answer—No!

To begin with, what need not be inevitable is the current practice of physicians in prescribing minor tranquilizers as a "quick" therapy for these stress-related or psychosomatic disorders. That approximately one hundred million prescriptions for minor tranquilizers were written in the United States alone last year attests to the magnitude of this practice. Unfortunately, drugs only partially extinguish the blaze once it has been kindled, and at the same time they frequently encourage the user, through symptom relief, to take on even more stress.

This begins a vicious cycle where even more drugs are needed to deal with even the routine conflicts of life, thus significantly impairing our innate potential for personal growth.

What are the alternatives to drugs? This chapter will present an overview of a number of popular techniques, all encouraging self-responsibility for health on the part of the person rather than responsibility for illness on the part of a physician.

As a background for discussing these techniques, we are aware that individuals highly trained in yoga techniques can indeed control bodily processes involving stress illnesses that were previously considered to be involuntary. Unfortunately, until the last decade, these demonstrations exerted relatively little practical influence on Western thinking, very likely because of the imagined rigors and mysticism involved in yoga training. Yet as early as 1906, William James (1960) began speculation about the potential power of the body to heal itself through similar self-regulation techniques:

> "I wonder whether the Yoga discipline may not be, after all, in all its phases, simply a methodical way of *waking up deeper levels of will power than are habitually used,* and thereby increasing the individual's vital tone and energy. I have no doubt whatever that most people live, whether physically, intellectually or morally, in a very restricted circle of their potential being. They *make use* of a very small portion of their possible consciousness, and of their soul's resources in general, much like a man who, out of his whole bodily organism, should get into a habit of using and moving only his little finger. Great emergencies and crises show us how much greater our vital resources are than we had supposed."

What an astounding insight! Why has it taken us so long to explore these new dimensions for both health care and personal growth? Probably the best answer is that, prior to the introduction of biofeedback in the 1960s, Western scientists lacked a meaningful model for understanding the voluntary self-regulation of body functions achieved via yoga techniques. Biofeedback is like a mirror that permits us to observe a normally hidden body function so that we can learn to control it. Whereas yogis require years of contemplation in order to achieve this mirror-like observation capability, biofeedback uses an instrument not unlike a radio (where the signal comes from the body rather than a radio station) to provide such observation instantaneously. This parallel has been noted by Elmer and Alyce Green (1977) of the Menninger Foundation, who have published a book called, *Biofeedback: The Yoga of the West.*

Once we recognized the· mirror model of biofeedback, a whole series of developments began which provided new dimensions for health care, many extending beyond biofeedback itself. For example, a number of investigators began to restudy a variety of meditation, yoga, and relaxation techniques that offered promise as alternatives to the increasingly widespread use and abuse of minor tranquilizers for the alleviation of the discomfort and disability caused by stress related disorders. About this same time, the concept of holistic medicine formally emerged, with an emphasis on individual self-responsibility for preventing and recovering from illness. Many physicians, too, were developing an awareness of the limitations of traditional scientific medicine, which used surgery or drugs to alter the body while often neglecting the person—his or her personality, his or her memory, important interpersonal issues, and potential for personal growth.

Perhaps I can best contrast our new dimensions in health care with traditional medical approaches by presenting a vignette of an individual suffering from a tension headache problem, probably the most frequent medical complaint. Although the mechanism of tension headache involves the spasm or excessive contraction of the muscles covering the skull producing a head pain akin to a "charley horse" in the leg, we experience this pain as coming from within the head, and, not infrequently develop recurrent concerns that we are suffering from some sort of brain tumor.

Studies have shown that individuals suffering from stress-related disorders, such as tension headache, are excessive users of the traditional health care system. For example, it is not at all unusual for an individual with tension headaches of some twenty years' duration to have sought medical evaluation in most major medical centers in the country annually or more often—seeking reassurance that he or she does not have cancer. The cost for this repetitive pattern of reassurance is staggering in comparison to alternative approaches discussed in this book, particularly in terms of misallocation of the resources of the existing expensive medical care system, in terms of personal suffering, and especially in terms of arrest in the growth potential of an individual whose life is focused on his pain.

Once a serious organic problem such as cancer has been ruled out, most physicians recognize that conscious or unconscious mental stress or anxiety is the basis for the symptom of head pain. Ideally, they would refer a tension headache patient to a psychologist or a psychiatrist, but through experience they have learned that most patients experiencing stress related pain reject such referral, feeling that the problem is not in their minds but entirely in their bodies—for their pain *is* very real. When such a referral is suggested the typical tension headache patient privately thinks to himself, "Doctor, you are the one who has something wrong with your head." As with psychotherapy, hypnosis can also be an effective treatment modality for stress related disorders, but the "cure" is often temporary, and most patients are fearful of the loss of control that the concept of hypnosis seems to imply to them. Hence, referrals for hypnotic treatment of the tension headache pain are usually rejected.

The most frequent "acceptable" alternative is to prescribe a minor tranquilizer, which tends to dampen the pathway from mental stress leading to excessive muscle contraction and tension headache pain.

In contrast to traditional medicine, holistic medicine emphasizes nondrug approaches, substituting voluntary self-regulation and self-responsibility for the involuntary dysregulation which produces the symptom. Whereas the typical tension headache patient will reject a referral to a psychiatrist, he is more likely to accept a referral to a biofeedback clinic where, through instrumentation, he can privately recognize the mental images and processes that increase the tension of his head muscles. The biofeedback instrument as a muscle tension mirror permits the individual to experience firsthand the mental activities which are contributing to excessive tension states. It is not unusual for a tension headache patient to experience marked reduction in headache frequency and intensity after six to ten hours of self-learning experience while attached to a biofeedback instrument. This is in marked contrast to the enormous expense of drugs and the requirements for repeated re-evaluation as provided by the traditional medical system.

Common to most of the self-regulation techniques now being identified by holistic physicians is a somewhat oblique strategy for achieving relaxation states incompatible with the body stress responses.

Why oblique? The Western work ethic encourages high achievement through goal directed effort; the tension headache patient who is advised to "just relax" attempts to do so with the same intense effort that is producing the symptom itself. Often this makes the frequency and severity of headache pain even worse. Stress prone individuals, therefore, need an oblique strategy that helps them to achieve the passive state necessary for voluntary self-regulation. For example, the individual attached to the biofeedback instrument for the treatment of tension headache is *not* told to "just relax"; rather, the person is told to attend to a tone that reflects his or her muscle tension and "to simply let the tone decrease through whatever mental images you find effective." Any direct strategy that encourages the person to try harder only serves to worsen the problem.

Further clarification of this difference between active and passive strategies is important. Healthy individuals exhibit a capacity to cope effectively with stressors, usually regaining a relaxed state within a relatively short time after "emergency response" episodes. This inherent quieting response allows their bodies to restore needed energy reserves, thus preparing them for subsequent arousal periods. On the other hand, persons who are predisposed to stress illnesses generally recover a state of relaxed balance much more slowly, if at all. Instead, they tend to maintain excessively high levels of activity in both muscle and hormonal systems. Although many biological factors—such as organic disease, tissue damage, or hostile environmental conditions—may contribute to such a recovery deficit, most stress prone individuals seem to gradually learn to override their inherent relaxation mechanisms. We are observing, for example, that children suffering from tension headache problems can reacquire this relaxed state much more readily than can adults who have had a longer history of exposure to stress. Eventually, the arousal response in adults apparently can become routinized, so that it has all the characteristics of an acquired, seemingly automatic, behavior pattern, one which the person comes to regard as "normal." Under such conditions the concepts of relaxation or calm lose their real meaning. Either the person reports that these states are elusive, often contending that they really should be avoided if "one is to make the most of life" or claiming to achieve them when body sensors indicate otherwise. In fact, sufferers of stress disorders frequently experience discomfort when they later achieve genuine physiological relaxation, suggesting how deeply ingrained their "stress expectancies" have become.

In summary, a common thread among self-regulation techniques is the creation of a state of passive alertness, a sense of looking within that cannot be achieved by trying too hard. The ancient Chinese philosopher, Lao Tzu (1944) captured the essence of this inner awareness which opens new vistas for body balance and personal growth as follows:

> There is no need to run outside
> For better seeing,
> Nor to peer from a window. Rather abide
> At the center of your being;
> For the more you leave it, the less you learn.
> Search your heart and see
> If he is wise who takes each turn:
> The way to do is to be.

SPECIFIC TECHNIQUES FOR
VOLUNTARY SELF-REGULATION
OF STRESS

We can view tension and stress as keeping us perched on a precipice of a barren mountain that seemingly becomes ever more menacing from the anxiety and pain of symptoms. From experiences with a variety of self-regulation techniques, I personally believe there are a variety of effective pathways down from the mountain to the tranquility of the more balanced conditions in the valley below.

Self-regulation techniques currently in widespread application as discussed in this chapter are passive meditation (Transcendental Meditation or TM, the derivative Relaxation Response [RR of Benson], and the derivative Clinically Standardized Meditation [CSM of Carrington]), progressive relaxation, autogenic training, biofeedback training, and the Quieting Response that I have developed.

Passive Meditation

Although yoga techniques have always fascinated Western man as paths to voluntary self-regulation, they have been resisted because of the imagined rigors and mysticism involved in them. This picture changed dramatically with the introduction of Transcendental Meditation, TM, to the Western world by Maharishi Mahesh Yogi in the ·1960s. The TM technique is simple, requiring four to six hours of verbal instruction and initial practice; it is entirely mental and does not require physical exercise, special diets, or other ascetic demands, thus making it particularly compatible with Western lifestyles. The meditation technique consists of sitting passively with eyes closed twice a day and thinking to oneself a Sanskrit sound, or mantra, which is given to the meditator by a teacher of the technique. (Recently the public press has published a report suggesting that age to the nearest five years is the method used for assigning one of sixteen "secret" TM mantras.) A growing body of experimental data substantiates that experienced meditators can produce relatively specific, unique, and consistent physiological changes that are incompatible with stress responses and a variety of stress-related disorders. As the potential health benefits of TM became recognized, two derivative passive meditation techniques have come into increasingly widespread use. The first, developed by Dr. Herbert Benson (1974), is called the Relaxation Response (RR), which uses progressive muscle relaxation, quiet breathing, and repetition to oneself of the mantra, "one." The second is Dr. Patricia Carrington's Clinically Standardized Meditation (CSM) (1978) which permits the beginning meditator to experiment and self select his own mantra from a list of sixteen Sanskrit mantras.

Although comparative studies seeking to evaluate the relative merits of the above three similar procedures are currently underway, the TM organization reportedly has become reticent about exposing its technique to further scientific investigation. This is likely to have the effect of encouraging more widespread adoption of one of the derivative procedures, such as RR or CSM.

Progressive Relaxation

Progressive relaxation is a technique developed by Edmund Jacobson (1978) in the 1920s which helps individuals contrast the difference between extreme muscle tension and complete relaxation of muscles progressively moving from one region of the body to another. This practice permits finer and finer discrimination of the extreme muscle tension states that lead to stress disorders. Although progressive relaxation can be a very effective treatment modality both to enhance health and to minimize problems such as tension headache, particularly when taught by a charismatic instructor over a period of many months, many patients view progressive relaxation by itself as being somewhat simplistic. It is apparently outside of the belief structure of Western man that progressive tensing and relaxing of body muscles could lead to the alleviation of symptoms.

However, almost everyone can identify with the sensation of

"bracing against" pain, for example, when one is in a dental chair and the dentist has not achieved adequate local anesthetic block of pain sensations. But enhanced awareness of this bracing effort, which is a common feature of almost all pain syndromes and has been studied extensively for twenty-five years by Whatmore (1974) (who describes it as "faulty effort" or dysponesis) has been incorporated in some derivative form into almost all types of voluntary self-regulation training strategies.

Autogenic Training

Autogenic training was a technique developed in Europe by Schultz (1959) early in this century, and it has subsequently been elaborately researched and popularized by Wolfgang Luthe (Schultz and Luthe, 1959). Autogenic training uses postures, exercises, and a set of standardized phrases (e.g., "My hands feel warm") which are autosuggestive in nature to help individuals gain voluntary self-regulation over a variety of body organ systems with practice. These autogenic phrases tend to emphasize the concepts of feelings of warmth and heaviness in the body.

The painstaking research efforts carried out by Dr. Luthe and his colleagues have established an extensive data base of indications, nonindications, and contraindications for self-regulation techniques that are likely to be applicable in all forms of self-regulation training. Unfortunately, optimal results with autogenic training require frequent contact with highly trained practitioners of this technique; because of the professional expense and time necessary to achieve autogenic control of dysregulated stress response symptoms, the technique *per se* has not been widely adopted in America. On the other hand, derivatives of autogenic training and its crucial and extensive data base are becoming widely recognized by practitioners of holistic medicine.

One promising method has been developed by Dr. Lester Fehmi based on applying autogenic phrases to the concept of space. Called Open Focus, it is a series of exercises on cassettes designed to assist the development of an open, relaxed and integrated mind-body state, in which focused awareness can be diffused to ultimately include the totality of on-going experience.

The goal is to develop a series of "objectless images" which facilitates the distribution of attention between and among various sensations and regions of the body and various types of experience. A series of questions designed to stimulate the imagination of objectless experience is typically represented by one question, "Can you imagine the distance or space between your eyes?" This enables one to approach relaxation as effortlessly as possible as opposed to narrow focus of attention which requires effort and tension to exclude other events and concentrate on one or a few.

Fehmi has interesting results in conjunction with E.E.G. (electroencephalographic) biofeedback training indicating balance and control of brainwaves is achieved during these training sessions.

Biofeedback

Biofeedback is a self-regulation technique with considerable appeal to Western man because of its use of instrumentation and its dramatic ability to demonstrate to a trainee the presence of unconscious tension states in different organ systems in the body. Biofeedback as a principle was identified and subsequently popularized by Kamiya (1969), Miller (1969), Brown (1970) and others and is now being pursued in research and clinical applications by over 2,000 members of the Biofeedback Society of America.

In contrast to our conscious awareness of the five senses and the extensive feedback from the skeletal muscles, functional reporting at the conscious level from smooth muscles and glands is meager, except under conditions of malfunction. The major feedback signal accompanying malfunction of these systems is the relatively crude sensation of pain sometimes referred to a distant location in the body.

The basic scientific principle of biofeedback is to provide parallel information via an external signal so that an inner body function becomes observable at the conscious level. This is accomplished with suitable sensors (electrical, thermal, and pressure, electronics and audiovisual or tactile feedback signals) that make the normally involuntary function available to the conscious brain so that it may use its capacity for learning to acquire voluntary control.

Some body systems have extensive feedback reporting to the conscious brain while others do not. A simple example will make this point clear. As part of the standard neurological examination a patient is asked to close his eyes, and to touch the left index finger to the tip of his nose. Most individuals perform this exercise with ease, using extensive feedback as to the position of the finger and the nose, carrying out differential calculus in three dimensions in order to complete the task satisfactorily.

This apparently unconscious feat which most of us take for granted could not be carried out by the world's fastest modern computer with the speed of our own brains. In contrast, if the same person is asked to pass a wave of contraction down his lower colon, he is unable to do so. In other words, we are relatively unaware of gastrointestinal activity, of blood pressure, of the mechanics of the heart, of the regulation of smooth muscle in our arteries—the "involuntary" inner machinery of the body—except when significant malfunction occurs. Although we are normally unaware of the automatic regulation of inner mechanisms, biofeedback permits us to acquire such control when corrections are needed. As an aside, it is probably fortunate that we do not normally have to use voluntary control of this inner body machinery, for if we were to have to consciously decide when to open or close each heart valve, or when to increase blood pressure in order to prevent fainting when changing body position, or when to pass a wave of contraction along the intestine in order to promote digestion, we would have no time left to carry out the unique intellectual functions— as well as others—that characterize the potential richness of human life.

Professor Neal Miller (1969), a pioneer in these studies, has speculated that:

Biofeedback should be well worth trying on any symptom, functional or organic, that is under neural control, that can be continuously monitored by modern instrumentation, and for which a given direction of change is clearly indicated medically . . . for example, cardiac arrhythmias, spastic colitis, and asthma, and those cases of high blood pressure that are not essential compensation for kidney damage.

To support Miller's speculation, the Biofeedback Society of America began a critical self-evaluation effort using thirty-five separate study sections (Biofeedback, 1977) to evaluate those applications of biofeedback for the treatment of stress related disorders deemed efficacious as compared to traditional medical treatment. Specific treatment applications of biofeedback currently judged most promising are for conditions of migraine headache, tension headache, neuromuscular reeducation following stroke and certain other types of neurological injury, fecal incontinence, primary Raynaud's syndrome (blanched fingertips, cold hands and feet due to inadequate blood flow), certain forms of sleep onset insomnia, and as an adjunct to psychotherapy and/or behavioral therapy for psychophysiological diagnoses. In the author's experience, the application of biofeedback *per se* to teach stress management and general relaxation is comparatively much less effective than passive meditative or other approaches. Using the same comparison, biofeedback is much more effective for the treatment of specific psychosomatic conditions.

An underlying issue here is that of long-term compliance with self-responsibility relaxation techniques. For general relaxation purposes we have observed the percentage of individuals continuing to practice three months after training is as follows: TM, 80%; Carrington's Clinically Standardized Meditation, 60%; Benson's Relaxation Response, 20%; combined electromyographic-thermal feedback for "general relaxation," 10% (Stroebel and Glueck, 1978). Investigations are currently underway to elucidate the roles of personality style, perceptual orienting style, hypnotic suggestibility, and the demand characteristics of each technique (very high for TM with its secrets and mystique, very low for biofeedback used for general relaxation). In contrast, compliance is very high for electromyographic-thermal biofeedback applied to *specific* psychosomatic problems in which symptom relief is self-reinforcing, as in the reduction of headache pain; compliance is much lower for conditions with relatively "silent" symptoms, such as hypertension.

Based on the issues of compliance and the self-reinforcing aspect of specific symptom relief, a number of investigators have differentiated potential applications of biofeedback into two categories: general stress reduction and specific treatment objectives. Non-biofeedback modalities with the best compliance, such as TM, are probably the techniques of choice for general stress reduction unless a fundamental change in attitude toward preventive medicine occurs, for example, reducing health insurance premiums for individuals who demonstrate continuing compliance with self-responsibility relaxation techniques.

Another alternative would be an acquisition program incorporating biofeedback and features of other self-regulation techniques, based on well-established principles of learning and reinforcement. This has been accomplished in Quieting Response Training, where trainees are initially asked the question, "Would six months be a reasonable period of time for you to acquire automatic skills in typing at a keyboard without looking at the keys?" The answer is invariably "Yes." To which the instructor responds, "Learning an automatic Quieting Response is no different. Will you agree to make a similar commitment to give yourself an automatic skill to achieve new dimensions in health and well being?"

The Quieting Response

While recognizing the widespread appeal and logic of biofeedback in providing an entree for busy Americans to gaining familiarity with the concept of self-responsibility for health care, I became concerned about the foregoing problems with low long-term compliance. I predicted that the potentials of biofeedback tor preventive medicine would likely not be realized unless a self-reinforcing technique were incorporated to ensure transfer of training outside of the initial learning setting with instruments attached. It was my observation that successful biofeedback subjects required between four and six months of regular practice of self-regulation skills before they developed a degree of automaticity in quieting that paralleled the inborn automaticity of the emergency response to stress.

What was needed was a quick mental mini-tranquilizer that could be elicited automatically while encountering mental stress and that would preclude inappropriate activation of bodily distress. Modern man, facing more frequent mental and less physical conflict, coupled with an intricate system of symbolic representation called language and an oftentimes rich fantasy life, has increasingly begun to activate his body's emergency responses inappropriately with regard to time, place, and person. The "red alert" emergency response for protection against real danger to the body is a protective system provided via genetics; the "pink alert," or even the "white alert,"—that is, imagined stresses or threats, are not.

Careful analysis of the physiology of the initial six to eight seconds of the stress response led to the formulation of a contrary Quieting Response that is triggered by annoyances and/or alterations in the breathing rhythm. After initial training to produce the sensations of limpness, warmth, and heaviness (training that is enhanced if accompanied by biofeedback) the six second Quieting Response is taught according to a learning curve concept in order to facilitate transfer of relaxation skills into all possible real life situations.

After four to six months of practicing the six second Quieting Response sixty to one-hundred times a day, whenever an annoyance is encountered, the low arousal state of reduced skeletal and smooth muscle tension can be achieved by most subjects within several seconds, even with the eyes open and while carrying on fairly normal type "A" behavior. This technique is in marked contrast to passive meditation procedures, which require two fifteen minute quiet periods each day. Many subjects fail to adhere to this twice daily practice schedule, which may explain why they stop the passive meditation technique.

An important component of the Quieting Response Training Program that reinforces frequent daily practice of the response is the computer scored *Psychophysiological Diary* (Stroebel, Luce, and Glueck, 1971), which is completed on a daily basis over the six-month training period, thus enhancing an individual's awareness of the body and mental factors contributing to distress related sensations. The computer scored *Diary* output is sensitive to trends and cycles in behavior leading to stress symptoms resulting from daily activities, activities that are normally forgotten by individuals as they encounter the pressures of each new day. In short, the computer's memory is used to help the person understand the role of daily activities in producing body distress.

The eight hour Quieting Response Training Program, which has already been incorporated into two thousand centers using biofeedback training, emphasizes the importance of coupling the hardware-instrumentation aspect of biofeedback with "software" instructions that aid in transfer of skills to real life situations. Individuals who privately purchase biofeedback instrumentation without understanding the importance of software in achieving biofeedback results have almost universally been disappointed in achieving control of stress problems.

My colleagues and I have observed an interesting *mental restructuring* in the way individuals permit stress to affect them as they acquire automaticity in eliciting the Quieting Response. Subjects report a new openness of mind, a sense of unity of body and mind, increased desire to give to and to help others, a greater thirst for knowledge, and, possibly most important, a sense of inner peace. This restructuring of mind-body perceptions creates a state of awareness and readiness for personal growth and for the achievement of greater self-actualization, as envisioned by other authors in this book.

SUMMARY

By tradition, the treatment of illness has been the focus of scientific medicine. It is true that once tissue damage has occurred, whether through infection, trauma, poison, congenital defect, or tumor, external intervention by modern medicine to patch the defect is impressive and often beyond the subjective control of the patient. However, the prevention and/or the onset of illness and our reactions to it are clearly not beyond personal control. These cannot be the private domain of the physician but are a matter of responsibility for each individual. Accustomed as he is to being a recipient rather than a participant in treatment, modern man apparently requires personal demonstration through a structured period of self-learning in order to incorporate the concept of self-responsibility into his daily lifestyle in times of both health and illness. Although this learning may best be accomplished at early ages, for example, with the teaching of the *four* Rs in the second grade— reading, 'riting, 'rithmetic, and *relaxation*—it is now accessible to all of us at any stage in life.

The remarkable degree of body control achieved through voluntary self-regulation techniques argues that man *need not be the inevitable victim of stress related illnesses.* Quite to the contrary, we have cited practical procedures now available for achieving the ever new vistas of our unrecognized vital resources for personal growth, as already envisioned by William James. To quote Karl Menninger (1959), these techniques can afford an opportunity to become even "healthier than healthy."

One of the keys to reaching a heightened sense of awareness of our inner resources is meditation. It enables a person to relate to productive self-regulatory mechanisms that provide a link to one's own higher self. Throughout time, meditation consistently appears in the writings and teachings of the mystics, religious prophets, and philosophers.

In recent years, many Westerners have looked to the Eastern philosophies, adopting many of the Eastern techniques and teachings in order to develop intuitive sensitivity. Others find those methods to be alien to their Western traditions and difficult to understand. The process of contemplation, however, is very much a part of the Old and New Testaments and is inherent in our heritage. It has been forgotten, or submerged, but it can form the basis of a Western-oriented quest for a knowledge of inner things, supported by historical and scientific experience.

Most meditative practices are somewhat less structured than some of the methods described by Dr. Stroebel. Meditation involves a more open-focused approach to relaxation. It is a personal experience that cannot be easily described. In some cases, it has produced various altered states of consciousness.

Dr. Abdullah outlines his valuable clinical experience with meditative processes and their beneficial effects in re-establishing harmony and balance. It may be one of the most important steps toward learning to cope with stress and changing one's perception. It is an integral part of man's search for fulfillment and self-actualization.

5

Meditation: Achieving Internal Balance

SYED ABDULLAH, M.D.

Meditation is a practice that moves the consciousness gradually toward a more holistic and serene state, opening up the higher spiritual faculties. When done systematically, and with dedication, meditation often produces remarkable changes in physiological states.

Meditation is primarily a journey into the inner self, with the aim of spiritual growth and a deeper maturity. It has no identity with any religion or dogma, although the higher forms of all the religions require meditation and contemplation as the direct path to spiritual development.

The spiritual path is seen as a cleansing from the concerns of the earth, from this life, enabling us to function "on the earth, but not of it." While bringing us into harmony with God, it achieves a therapeutic value by cutting through our anxieties relating to illusions of security and problems of interpersonal relations.

Many forms of meditation exist; each is suited to different

people in different cultures at different times in the history of man. The form is not relevant. The process is. Whatever method is chosen, the practice should lead—when done with discipline and dedication to higher purpose—to a greater inner awareness that produces an experience of greater peace for the individual.

These spiritual considerations should be seen as primary in any discussion of meditation. Mystics have long known of meditation's therapeutic effects but have never considered the therapeutic function as central to its purpose. It is only in recent years in the West and in some scientific establishments in India that meditation has been assessed as a therapeutic tool. Research on the technique has by now reached considerable proportions, and there is a need to begin collecting and synthesizing the relevant information on its potential in self-healing. In that respect, it is a potent force.

John A. Sanford (1977), in one interpretation of meditation, describes it as ". . . working with an image. Psychological meditation uses an image that has come from one's own unconscious. In meditation the image interacts with the conscious personality in such a way that both are changed. The result is a modification of the conscious standpoint in favor of the unconscious, and a gradual assimilation of the unconscious into the ego structure. In this way, images and symbols from the unconscious are used by the transforming function of the symbols."

Sanford's description of meditation is one of many insights and interpretations of a subject as old as man himself. It can be seen as a generalized word having to do with any quiet process that puts us into tune with our unconscious and leads us further into our deeper spiritual states. In many respects, meditation has no limits to its depths, no limits to its possibilities for the development of humankind.

Some see it as any disciplined activity engaged in by the mind—that is, any activity centered on a goal. That definition, however, may be too sweeping. Meditation's goal is to achieve spiritual oneness, the highest expression of an integrated personality. Consciously or not, its process is directed toward that.

Once one starts in meditation, the path to growth is unavoidable and is not always comfortable. For to reach the sense of God requires the eradication of illusions. That is what happens in meditation.

This chapter will not discuss the mystical aspects of meditation but will instead describe some high points of research and treatment that have used meditation in a Western medical setting.

Meditation's well-known calming effects on the central nervous system and on the autonomic nervous systems are often quite dramatic, leading to extensive application in treating the self for overcoming the many stress-related and anxiety-related disorders so prevalent in contemporary society. It is particularly effective in handling emotional disturbances because of its effectiveness in tapping into the centers of our self and thus controlling anxiety and related psychophysiological disorders.

It is thus a useful adjunct to psychotherapy in providing a relatively direct approach to a person's unconscious. The mental images evoked in the process can be utilized in much the same way as dream material is handled in conventional therapy.

Therapists and researchers see meditation as an essentially psychological maneuver aimed at altering the ordinary status of human consciousness in order to obtain certain therapeutic objectives. Experiencing, if only temporarily, an anxiety-free state is perhaps the most immediate reward of meditation. In this calmer, more serene state, the individual's consciousness is free to drift toward his more creative and spiritual potentialities.

The research done by Wallace and Benson (1972) has shown that the shift in the psychological profile of the individual is clearly toward a quiet, restful state of body and mind. Brain waves and pulse rate slow down, respiration becomes slower and deeper, oxygen consumption and carbon dioxide excretion go down (indicating a decrease in metabolic rate), muscle tension decreases as the muscles relax, and both the electrical resistance of the skin and the circulation of the blood within its vessels increase. These and other changes suggest that the involuntary nervous system dominates voluntary pathways during meditation.

Benson (1975) has evolved a simplified version of meditation that is effective in alleviating mild and moderate forms of essential hypertension. He has also proposed that human beings have a capacity to invoke a state of relaxation response that is the exact opposite of the well-known "flight or fight" response.

In emotionally excitable states, the heart rate, cardiac output, and the narrowing of the blood vessels of the kidney all lead to an increase in the blood pressure. The toning down of the sympathetic nervous system and the emotional calming produced by meditation, according to Benson (1975), have beneficial effects on hypertension, and several investigators have corroborated these findings. For example, lowering of the enzyme known as dopamine beta-hydroxylase and a decrease of the renin activity in the blood during meditation further point to the far-reaching effects of this simple procedure on factors affecting blood pressure. (Renin is the substance released by the kidney and is one agent responsible for an increase in blood pressure.) Although it has not assumed the place of the primary therapy for hypertension, meditation's adjunctive role appears to be highly promising.

Other stress-based disorders such as colitis, migraine, tension headaches, and menstrual cramps often show spontaneous remissions or amelioration during the regular practice of meditation. Many people suffering from chronic insomnia find relief in meditating while lying in bed. Further, the sleep produced in this manner seems to be more refreshing than that obtained by sleeping pills, and there are none of the adverse aftereffects of medication.

There have also been anecdotal reports of the beneficial effects of meditation on epilepsy and cardiac arrhythmias, although further studies of a critical nature must be done before these claims can be authenticated.

More commonly, improvement in many chronic skin conditions has been noted in association with regular meditation. Acne, pimples, dryness of skin, and some forms of eczema respond favorably even when they are not the specific goal of treatment. Perhaps the combination of the improved peripheral circulation and the increased electrical resistance of the skin bring about these nonspecific beneficial effects. An as yet untested but highly important hypothesis is that during meditation, the hormonal balance of the body improves, since it is mediated by the hypothalamus, where meditation makes its fundamental physiological impact. This might be an added factor in the skin improvements so often noted.

One patient, a fifty-three-year-old woman, was being treated for asthma by a simple breathing exercise and meditation. Her atopic eczema, from which she had suffered since childhood, cleared up in the course of the treatment. As the patient learned to develop control over her bronchial spasms, she began to hope for and visualized an improvement in her skin condition. Her body's healing processes are likely to have come into play in the meditative state. She had been on steroids for many years, but she gradually discontinued them without any flare-up in the skin condition. Follow-up after a year and a half showed the skin to be free of any leisons.

The stress emotions, aroused under situations of real or imagined threat to the organism, are essential parts of the adaptive process of the body. However, when the stress factors assume a chronic quality, these same adaptive mechanisms can contribute to illness. Stress reactions are meant to aid in short-term emergency situations, during which they act less harmoniously in order to serve the total physiological needs of the body. If this state is continued over an extended period of time, psychosomatic illnesses appear that may produce permanent tissue damage, cause more stress, and thereby perpetuate the vicious cycle. The timely use of the relaxation-meditation exercises tends to minimize these stress reactions, to activate the relaxation response, and to foster healing in the stressed organ systems.

Simonton has described elsewhere in this book (see Chapter 6) some success in the treatment of cancer patients with the combined use of meditation and imagery, and there have been other reports of the beneficial effects of this approach when combined with the established methods of treatment. Most of these reports have been of anecdotal nature and await further authentication, but they seem most promising. Meares reports, in the *Medical Journal of Australia* (1976), the regression of cancer in both breasts of a forty-nine-year-old woman with the use of what he terms "intensive meditation." Her cancer was pathologically established, and there was radiological evidence of its spread to the spine. The writer states that, whatever the final outcome, her condition underwent a dramatic change for the better, a change that was much more than the relief of pain and an improved state of mind. He theorizes that some cancers are related to the immunological reactions, and there is a similarity between the immunological and allergic reactions. Moreover, some cancers are influenced by endocrine reactions. Meares suggests that the beneficial effect seen in his patient might be explained by the fact that meditation may modify the hormonal as well as the allergic reactions of the body.

After studying the techniques of spiritual healers for many years, LeShan (1974) has developed a comprehensive course in healing techniques through meditation. In his view, a state of "clairvoyant reality" is reached in the healing meditative process, during which there is a merging of the therapist, the patient, and the universe. LeShan also contends that psychic healing skills can be acquired by anyone who is willing to go through the rigors of disciplined training in meditation. LeShan himself uses a wide variety of meditative techniques, and each trainee is encouraged to adopt the method that he or she prefers. He does not insist on the practice of mystical-spiritual modalities, believing that the healing art can be taught as a discipline in itself. He does, however, mention that the act of healing brings about spiritual growth in the healer.

In LeShan's approach to the use of meditation, the patient generally assumes a passive role. Indeed, Leshan claims that it is not even necessary for the patient to be informed about the process. He emphasizes that psychic healing should be restricted to the position of an adjunct to the accepted forms of treatment provided by qualified physicians.

During meditation, the patient can make himself become more intensely aware of his bodily functions. The awareness of the breath, of muscular tensions, and of visceral movements can easily be increased by the simple procedure of passive attention. This acts as a natural feedback system, and it has been used in some mystical orders to teach control of the automatic functions of the various organ systems. Biofeedback techniques are essentially based on this principle, except that electronic monitoring devices of brain waves and muscle tension expedite the process and make it more predictable and repeatable.

Recent studies (Galin and Ornstein, 1972; Galin, 1974; Sperry, 1964, 1968) on the left and right hemispheres of the brain have significantly added to the scientific understanding of what happens in meditation. The two halves of the brain look alike and are the same in size, weight, metabolism, and cellular structure. Studies done so far enable us to draw a tentative profile of the dominant and the nondominant modes of consciousness. The left hemisphere, which is dominant in the right-handed person, is responsible for the verbal, analytic, logical, and intellectual modes of consciousness. It processes information in a lineal sequential manner, like the sentences on this page, and is aware of the sense of time.

This is the action mode, concerned with the manipulation of the environment in the service of survival-related tasks. It has priority in the use of the motor and sympathetic nervous systems. Since it deals with contingencies related to fight or flight, anxiety is its natural emotional component.

The right hemisphere, on the other hand, is nondominant and subserves the more receptive mode of consciousness that processes multiple stimuli simultaneously, transforming them into wholes. Unlike its dominant counterpart, this mode of consciousness tends to be nonverbal, spatial, tacit, and diffuse. It is more intuitive and inspirational than logical. It has little control over the muscular and sympathetic systems, and it depends on the dominant hemisphere for the execution of its drives.

Not being directly involved in the struggle for survival, the right hemisphere's physiological profile is of a low arousal, parasympathetic type. Most of our waking life is spent in the left hemispheric mode, and our chief educational emphasis is on the cultivation of the faculties of this side. The left side receives constant reinforcements by way of creature comforts and other material rewards, while the right hemispheric mode of consciousness is by and large left to its own devices.

In their wisdom, the mystical traditions have always emphasized that there is more to human consciousness than is manifested in the left hemisphere state of goal-oriented striving. The right hemisphere and its methodical development have been their chief concern. Their approach has been subjective and experiential, and the use of meditation in one form or another is a central theme. The active mode of being is suspended during meditation, and so are the logical, analytic ways of thinking. A sense of timelessness, a dissolution of sharp ego boundaries, and a feeling of oneness with the universe are produced in advanced states of meditation. During these moments, there is a resolution of inner conflicts and an absence of anxiety. In effect, the left hemispheric mode is held in abeyance and the nondominant mode is cultivated. In this way, the disciple is gradually made ready to receive the highest universal teachings.

It appears that in the clinical use of meditation this same reversal of the hemispheric dominance is achieved, although to a lesser degree. The physiological accompaniments of this state are then utilized for therapeutic purposes. Although this may be regarded as a way of using a higher technique for a more circumscribed purpose, on occasions, a patient may experience a genuine breakthrough of spiritual insight.

For example, a patient of mine, who was being treated for hypertension by a relaxation-meditation technique, reported to me that while meditating at home, she had an experience of God. This was particularly surprising to her, since she had always been an atheist. Now, at the age of sixty-five, she felt a loosening from a set of "logical" ways of thinking and became aware of an orderliness and meaning in life that unexpectedly released her from all her neurotic anxieties. It is to be noted that in her therapy sessions, the subject of God was never raised, the goal of treatment being merely the control of hypertension.

A widow and mother of two grown children, she was alone and about to retire from her job. Her loneliness at this point in her life was compounded by her fear of getting a stroke. With this single mystical experience, all these concerns lost their crippling quality, her blood pressure normalized, and she developed a healthy optimistic attitude toward the future. She became a source of strength and emotional support to her children and friends, and she discovered many creative ways of spending her time in retirement.

Although she was hard put to describe the oceanic feeling of ecstasy that had engulfed her when she felt that "experience of Divine presence," she remained sure that "everything was going to be all right." She also discovered that she had lost the fear of dying. Two years after therapy was terminated, she continues to meditate, her blood pressure continues to be normal, and she has retained a joyful attitude toward life and what lies beyond it. She has developed into an intensely spiritual person and is still in the process of growth.

This case, by no means an isolated one, shows the potentially powerful impact of the meditative approach—even when such an impact is not the explicit goal. The simple act of suspending the left cerebral mode of consciousness can sometimes open up one's heretofore unrecognized faculties, making a person aware of many alternatives available to him, alternatives of which he was previously unaware.

Meditation can serve as a valuable aid to the process of psychotherapy. The appearance of flashes of memory, images out of the unconscious, unexplained emotional experiences, and physical sensations during meditation are well known. Sensations of touch, taste, changes in temperature, abdominal cramps, and the like are also reported. These experiences, when explored in the course of psychotherapy, sometimes provide valuable clues. Hypnogogic images are particularly useful in the exploration of the patient's deeper consciousness as the patient is encouraged to talk about them. These images are used in the same way as dream material. The advantage is that this material can be obtained almost on demand, and the recall is usually much more complete and reliable.

One patient, while meditating, saw a play of green colors, followed by the outline of a human figure stooping to pick up a child and hold him tenderly in his arms. The patient could not recognize the figures, either of the adult or the child, but remembered that the adult was wearing a white garment with a high neck. When asked to associate to that image, he mentioned that his father on his recent visit from California gave him a green turtleneck shirt. It will be noted that in the meditation the unknown adult was wearing a white turtleneck, the green color having shifted to the background. His next association was how as a child he hated his father's body odor and always avoided having anything to do with his clothes. The shirt in question was purchased by the father for himself, but after wearing it once he found it too tight and decided to give it to his son. It was a measure of the lessening of his hostile feelings toward his father that the patient was able to accept and wear the shirt.

In the course of therapy, the patient had worked through most of his conflicts toward his father and had become aware of an urge to cultivate closeness with the aging man. The father's visit from California was in response to his invitation. The reconciliation between the father and son was symbolically ratified during meditation by the vision of the little child being embraced by an adult wearing a turtleneck. It appears that the meditation imagery helped the patient tie in the fragments of past and present experiences and regard his relationship with the father more positively.

Another patient, while meditating, noticed that his feet had become tense, although the rest of his body was relaxed. I asked him to "get in touch" with the tightness in his feet and to search for associations. After a long pause, the patient said, "The only thought that comes to my mind is my father telling me that I will never amount to anything." I then asked him how this could be related to the tightness in his feet. There was another pause, and then the patient went on, "I remember his saying that I will never be able to stand on my own two feet." After having said this, the patient noticed a marked easing of the tension in his feet.

A female patient noticed bitter tastes in her mouth while meditating. She associated this to the bitter taste of a stuff her parents used to paint on her thumb to prevent her from thumb-sucking. She cried bitterly as she related to me the humiliation she suffered when her painted thumb became the object of ridicule at school. Perhaps this painful memory would not have been uncovered had it not been for the bitter taste the patient experienced during meditation. The nonverbal cue thus became very helpful in understanding an important factor in her dynamics.

Another technique often helpful in psychotherapy, I have found, is to ask the patient to actively visualize scenes, such as the faces of significant persons in his life, rather than to wait for images to appear spontaneously. For example, one patient related a violent quarrel he had with his wife when she had accidentally broken a cologne bottle in the bathroom. His reaction to this seemingly minor event was disproportionately severe, and he had passed an entire week arguing with her about it. Sensing it to be symbolically significant, I asked the patient to visualize the face of his mother while he meditated. On coming out of the meditative state, he recalled a long-forgotten incident from his childhood when his mother had tried to make him sip her urine from a bottle into which she had just voided. Reportedly, this was to cure him of a chest ailment. As he refused to do so, the mother forced the bottle to his mouth, a scuffle ensued in which the bottle fell to the floor, and the foul-smelling urine spread over the floor.

From this association, it was easy enough for the patient to see the symbolic relationship between the two events. He was also able to gain insights into several aspects of his marital conflicts. The immediate effect was the relief of the intense anger he had been feeling toward his wife over this particular incident.

During such moments of insight, there can be an opening

up of the floodgates of the unconscious, presenting a wealth of important data and a great challenge to the patient and to the therapist. From my experience, I know that the therapist must intervene promptly and skillfully in order to channel and contain these outpourings within the limits of the patient's capacity to assimilate them. This requires full familiarity with the patient's psychodymanics and psychopathology. Otherwise, there is danger of confusion and disruption of the psychotherapeutic process. Without sufficient safeguards, an over-psychotic decompensation may be precipitated in vulnerable individuals.

Still other studies (Shafii, Lavely, and Jaffe, 1975; Benson and Wallace, 1972) suggest the value of meditation in handling drug abuse. It has been reported by several investigators that a large number of meditators have subsequently given up the use of drugs. It seems likely that drugs induce an altered state of consciousness that holds great fascination for those who find reality too burdensome. The altered state of consciousness produced by meditation, though not identical with that produced by drugs, may provide a similar relief. In view of its far greater safety, meditation has obvious advantages over drugs. Moreover, whereas the latter often produces fragmentation and disorganization of the personality, meditation leads to a harmonious growth and integration of the personality.

The marked lowering of anxiety during meditation also makes it a valuable tool in behavior therapy. A businessman with a phobia for high buildings, planes, and elevators was asked to visualize being on the eightieth floor of a building during a deeply relaxed meditative state. He was also instructed to report any spontaneous images that occurred. One of the images he reported was that of his father threatening to throw him out of the window. This session was the turning point in the treatment.

In subsequent sessions, he came to understand that his infantile fear of being thrown out of the window had colored his relationship with other men and had particularly restricted his effectiveness in dealing with aggressive adversaries in business.

To sum up, meditation opens up a rich inner resource that is almost inexhaustible. In some cases, easy oscillations between the conscious and the unconscious processes bring about that "magic synthesis" that is often conducive to creativity and to spiritual peak experiences. The individual may even become increasingly aware of alternatives available to him in his every-day purusits, as well as in his higher level activities.

In this chapter, I have focused primarily on the use of meditation in the therapeutic situation, choosing to leave to the other authors discussion of its power in self-healing. For the average person—that is, the only mildly neurotic individual—meditation as a self-assessment process and centering technique, as a form of spiritual growth, is to be highly recommended.

Meditation as self-therapy or as a daily practice can thus be an exciting and enriching adventure into one's inner self, an adventure in which one can afford to be absolutely honest in learning to look at oneself in the totality of experience.

We have considered two basic ways of viewing disease: to look for the pathogens and to examine the host resistance. Immunology in medical research has received considerably more attention in the past fifteen years. The focus has been on the role of the immune system—the body's natural defenses—in sickness and in health.

A growing number of clinicians are inclined to believe that development of a cancer does not require just the presence of abnormal cells but also requires some disturbance in the body's normal defenses.

Carl Simonton, a radiation oncologist (a physician specializing in the treatment of cancer), is one of those clinicians who believe that something is happening in the person who contracts the disease to create a susceptibility. He recognizes the strong link between stress and illness. In his Center, he and his wife (Stephanie Matthews–Simonton, Director of Counseling) see patients from all over the United States, most of whom have received a "medically incurable" diagnosis from their doctors. Their innovative methods rely heavily on the value of meditative processes and psychotherapy to help the patient participate in changing the dis-order in his life that contributed to the development of the malignancy.

6

Stress, Self-Regulation, and Cancer

O. CARL SIMONTON, M.D.
STEPHANIE MATTHEWS-SIMONTON

It is our decided opinion that a person's mental attitudes and his emotional make-up play a role both in the development of cancer and in the course of that disease. In our work at the Cancer Counseling and Research Center in Fort Worth, Texas, we attempt to alter the course of malignancy by addressing the emotions of the cancer patient.

We believe that cancer is often an indication of problems elsewhere in an individual's life, problems aggravated or compounded by a series of stresses six to eighteen months prior to the onset of cancer. The cancer patient has typically responded to these problems and stresses with a deep sense of hopelessness, or "giving up." This emotional response, we believe, in turn triggers a set of physiological responses that suppress the body's natural defenses and make it susceptible to producing abnormal cells.

The research and observations on psychological factors in cancer go back at least to the time of Galen, about the second century A.D. Galen said depressed women had a greater tendency to develop malignancy than happy women. The same sorts of factors were observed by physicians throughout the Dark Ages, the Middle Ages, the Renaissance, and the Victorian Era. In the 1950s came a surge of psychological studies attempting to link cancer with personality factors.

In 1971, Dr. Art Schmale completed psychological interviews with women who had questionable pap smears and who were about to have biopsies to establish whether they showed evidence of uterine cancer. Schmale was able to predict whether or not a woman was going to have a postive or negative biopsy with 73.6 percent accuracy. What he felt he was observing was a sense of hopelessness and helplessness in these women.

Three researchers, West, Blumberg, and Ellis (1952), used standard psychological tests to predict the course of malignancy. They were able to predict with 78 percent accuracy whether or not a person was going to have a fast- or slow-growing tumor, regardless of medical prognosis. What they were picking up on was impaired emotional outlets. The fewer emotional outlets a patient developed, the worse was his prognosis and the faster his growth rate of cancer.

The work of Dr. Caroline B. Thomas of Johns Hopkins Hospital (1974) is the most exciting to appear lately. Dr. Thomas started a longitudinal study thirty-one years ago and did structured interviews, along with psychological tests, on senior medical students at the Johns Hopkins University. She attempted to correlate psychological factors with five illnesses: heart disease, high blood pressure, cancer, suicide, and mental illness.

The group that was the most psychologically distinct was the group that had developed malignancy. The two primary observations she made that set them apart from the population as a whole were lack of closeness to parents and impaired emotional outlets. The fewer tools we've developed for communicating, the less healthy we tend to be.

To us, there are three concepts that are important in addressing the emotions of the cancer patient and in attempting to understand the disease.

The first is that of host resistance. Our previous understanding of malignancy was that it was a disease that developed for very vague reasons and that if a person was to regain his health, it was going to be through rapid dramatic intervention, such as surgery, chemotherapy, and radiation.

In the late 1960s we were presented with the basic underlying concept behind the widely accepted surveillance theory in the development of malignancy. That is, that we all develop cancer cells, that we're exposed to cancer-causing agents. We have anticancer mechanisms in us that recognize these cells and destroy them.

One part of the problem in the development of malignancy is that those natural host-resistant elements are not working normally. Bathrop (1977) has shown, in a study of recently widowed people, that the activity of their T-lymphocytes is depressed during the period of grief following loss. These concepts all interrelate intimately, as intimately as the relations between mind and body. But in the problem of overcoming malignancy, we have come to understand much more—that the ultimate ridding of our malignant cells depends on host resistance.

When we do surgery for an early breast cancer, we know that cancer cells are dislodged and that they circulate through the system; if those cells don't grow, that means that our basic host resistance destroyed those cells. Even with surgical incision, we know that cancer cells get dislodged.

With radiation therapy, we know that we hit only a certain number of cells, and when the amount is reduced to a small number of cells, the final destruction of malignancy depends on host resistance. So, the importance of focusing on host resistance is vital in looking at what the person can do in maintaining health and in overcoming malignancy.

The second concept is that of the role of chronic stress. We know that exposure to chronic stress increases the susceptibility to disease in general and to cancer in particular. Dr. Hans Selye has already outlined earlier in this book (see Chapters 2 and 3) the relationship of stress to disease. His early research formed the basis of the modern work on stress today. Of great importance in cancer work is his discovery that chronic stress suppresses the immune system, which is the mechanism responsible for engulfing and destroying cancerous cells or alien microorganisms.

The work of Solomon (1969) and Riley (1975) shows that when exposed to prolonged chronic stress, animal host resistance breaks down, increasing susceptibility to infectious diseases, to illnesses in general, and to malignancy in particular. The work of Holmes (1970) has shown that if we are exposed to increasingly stressful events, our susceptibility increases. And our susceptibility to disease increases in proportion to the amount of stress we experience.

Now, certainly there are individual differences, and there are problems with applying work that has been done on general populations to individuals. We can talk about these observations in general terms, but when we try to apply them to individual experiences, there are individual variations that cause them to perhaps become confusing. But we need to take them into account as we address these concepts, because stressful events to one person are not stressful events to another. We accordingly need to understand our patient and to get to know him in a different way than we did when we applied standard medical treatment. Both kinds of observation are appropriate within their dimension.

The third concept concerns the work done on biofeedback. Biofeedback was our avenue into the understanding that our thoughts and emotions influence body functions, and we began thinking of it as a tool to influence host resistance. We could also learn to use it to measure reaction to stressful events. Now we were beginning to appreciate a tool for interacting with the problem that was becoming increasingly clear in our own thinking. So we began to explore what biofeedback was, what its possibilities were for application; and we began to see similarities between biofeedback and hypnosis, self-hypnosis, various forms of meditation, autogenic training, Benson's (1975) regular relaxation response, and Jacobson's (1938) progressive relaxation. All involved a central quieting and a participation in the process.

As we appreciated how part of the problem in the development of malignancy was related to a breakdown in the immune system, we were elated with the possibility of using biofeedback in an attempt to correct that deficiency, to bring these mechanisms back to the normal state.

As we pursued these various forms of influencing host defenses, more and more commonalities began to appear. It also seemed that the person using biofeedback was interacting with a process that made sense to him. The woman with heart disease was in her own mind doing something that made sense to her and would influence her disease, and what she was doing tended to take the form of pictures. It made sense to us because we appreciated the interactions between thoughts and the emotional reactions that went with them, and at the same time recognized how these reactions influenced hormonal balance.

Endocrine balance, we knew, was important in controlling the production of malignant cells in laboratory conditions. Thus, it would seem that the more a person could take part in producing healthier emotions, the more his hormonal balance would swing toward normal. Thus, there would be less tendency for cancer cells to be produced in response to the number of cancer-producing agents, and the person's general health would be benefited.

So, in understanding the neurological connections, it seemed, from a straight psychological and physiological standpoint, that biofeedback and basic emotional understanding were potentially powerful tools for dealing with malignancy,

We then tried to come up with a procedure that we could explain to a patient. Carl first went over this process with his five-year-old daughter, and when it was clear and simple to her, we then felt ready to begin talking to our patients about it. The central theme seemed to be one of relaxation in which a patient would imagine what they wanted to happen. Three times a day was effective for this imaging, and we set a limit, from our own experience in biofeedback, of no less than five and no more than fifteen minutes for the process.

If we didn't take enough time, we found that the quieting process was not effective. If we took as long as we felt we needed, we never would stop, because we never got to an end point. We were trying to get the patient to picture regaining his health in a way that made sense to us and, I hoped, would make sense to him. We had to be honest about what was going on and to do it in a way that would make the patient feel comfortable.

We had him picture his cancer, the treatment he was getting, and the activity of the white blood cells. We had him picture white blood cells coming in and destroying the malignancy, had him see the treatment coming in—the radiation therapy—and hitting the cancer cells and destroying them in a way that worked as we understood it. We had him do this exercise three times a day. After he finished seeing the white blood cells destroy the cancer cells, he was then to picture himself regaining his health and his ability to eat a little better. He could image whatever he wanted.

The first patient had a very dramatic response. He was sixty-one years old and had an advanced throat cancer that was not previously treatable. He weighed only ninety-eight pounds when we began. We anticipated that he would get worse and die. He couldn't eat, and he could barely swallow his saliva. He very rapidly regained his health and had almost no side effects to treatment. He then used the process on his arthritis, and he overcame that as well as his sexual impotence, which he had also had for twenty years.

Very few subsequent patients, as it turned out, responded in the same way, but over time we were able to improve the technique with a deeper appreciation of the diversity and complexity of individuals and their malignancies.

One of the early things we found useful in helping patients to identify their participation in the onset of their disease was to ask them to identify the major stresses occurring in their lives six to eighteen months prior to their diagnosis. We used this list of stresses as a basis for discussing with the patients how they had participated in their illness by creating or allowing undue stresses in their lives or perhaps by refusing to recognize that they do have emotional limits. Some patients, we found, have subordinated their own needs to everybody elses', so that they have no strength left to devote to themselves. Others, we found, reacted to stresses with feelings of helplessness or hopelessness.

To give you a brief idea of some of the specifics we have just discussed, we ask patients to identify stresses in the six to eighteen months prior to their disease onset in the following way. We ask them to list, on paper, five major life changes or stresses that occurred in this time period. We find that when people begin to list such things, even if they do not identify major external stresses, they are usually able to find some internal stresses, such as some serious disappointment, a major change in a personal relationship, or some serious questioning of their self-identity. The object of this self-examination is to help the patient identify beliefs or behaviors they are exhibiting that they may wish to change. Because they have been listed as major stresses, they obviously have some threatening effect on the patient's health.

We find that as patients begin to look at their behavior and at themselves in more detail, they are more inclined to be willing to accept some role that they themselves play as a participant in the development of their cancer. Most of our patients begin to see important links between their emotional states and the onset of their disease.

It is extremely important that in this process the patient does not feel guilty in being asked to identify these kinds of behavior. We help them to understand that mistakes are always made and that the exercise is one of trying to understand their problems rather than one of placing blame on themselves for behavior they may have exhibited. The object of this self-exploration is also to help them find more effective means of coping with their stresses so that they may make more energy available with which to fight the disease.

We emphasize to them that it takes great courage to explore with understanding how they can change what they thought, as a result of family or cultural influences, was true about themselves. We congratulate them for their willingness to participate in the process of exploring their own emotions and attitudes and for being willing to reject those that are creating self-destruction.

We also find it helpful during the process of working with our patients to get them to identify five or more most important benefits they received from a major illness in their lives. This certainly does not suggest that people consciously select being sick. But the interesting thing we find is that the five areas listed most frequently are as follows:

1. Receiving permission to get out of dealing with a troublesome problem or situation.
2. Getting attention, care, and nurturing from people around them.
3. Having an opportunity to regroup their psychological energy to deal with a problem or to gain a new perspective.
4. Gaining an incentive for personal growth or for modifying undesirable habits.
5. Not having to meet their own or others' high expectations.

When patients identify the secondary gains from their illnesses, they learn what emotional needs it will be important to meet other than through illness, as they get well.

We have found that relaxation and mental imagery (some people know it as visualization techniques) are excellent tools to help people reinforce their beliefs in their ability to recover from cancer. We find that when the relaxation technique is practiced first, this enables them to learn the basic means of reducing tension and distractions so that they are then prepared physically to deal with the second phase, the mental imagery process.

The relaxation technique we have devised for our program is largely taken from Dr. Edmond Jacobson (1938), who developed the technique called "progressive relaxation." By learning to relax and to influence their bodies, people are able to accept their physical sensations once again and are reinforced in their recognition that they can control muscle tension. The relaxation also helps reduce fear, which, of course, can be overwhelming in life-threatening diseases like cancer.

We recommend to our patients that they do the relaxation exercises three times a day for ten to fifteen minutes each. This also includes the mental imagery. We give them a specific set of instructions in the form of a tape recording, allowing plenty of time for completing each step in the process.

Although relaxation is of great value, we would like to repeat that it is really a prelude to mental imagery, since it enables the person to reduce tension that might distract from concentrating on the imagery itself. The imagery exercises stem from Stephanie's background in motivational psychology. Her experiences made us conscious of the opportunity to alter the belief systems of people in different walks of life through different types of mind-control disciplines. The common thread connecting these various disciplines is that people create mental images of desired events.

By forming an image, a person makes a clear mental statement of what he wants to happen, and by repeating the statements, he or she comes to expect that the desired event actually will occur. The behavior of the person then begins to be consistent with the desired result. The image forming is really a self-fulfilling prophecy of a positive kind.

The steps we give our patients are designed to systematically take them from a state of sitting quietly in a room with soft lighting in a comfortable chair, through relaxing various muscles in parts of the body, to visualizing the cancer cells being destroyed either by treatments or by some other mental images. This is only a bare outline of the procedures, which are described in considerable detail in our book written with J. Creighton, *Getting Well Again* (1978).

Since we first used the visualization method in 1971, we have made it the central element in our program. Not only does this mental imagery process create changes in the patient's expectancy, but it also seems to have the side benefits of helping the patient discover parts of himself in other phases of his life.

We consistently direct our attention to the patient's belief systems, for we have found that such expressed or unexpressed feelings can have a significant influence on the onset and progress of cancer. This is true of other illnesses as well.

We have found that part of the stress and tension experienced by many patients is very often due to a difficulty in expressing negative feelings, particularly anger and resentment. Suppressing such negative feelings has the effect of increasing stress on the body and serving to inhibit recovery. Here also, it is important not to convey a feeling of teaching a person what they "ought" or "should" do, but rather to give them specific methods that they may use to relieve themselves of such feelings.

Among the many benefits of this relaxation/mental imagery process, two are significantly related to the process of self-regulation. First, the process serves as a method for appraising current belief systems and for altering those beliefs, if desired. Second, the process can affect physical changes, enhancing the immune system and altering the course of a malignancy. Since mental processes have a direct influence on the immune system and on hormonal balances on the body, we can attribute physical changes to changes in thought patterns.

It has been our policy not to accept patients unless they are accompanied by a spouse; if patients are unmarried, we ask that they bring their closest family member. On some occasions, we have worked with the son or brother or daughter or sister. We find that there are two important reasons for this firm policy. First, when patients are asked to begin changing their attitudes about their disease or to adopt mental imagery programs, the support of the family member becomes very important in helping the patient's regularity in carrying out the directions. Second, spouses or family members frequently need as much if not more support in helping to cope with their own feelings about the disease.

During Carl's specialty training at medical school, he was always curious about why certain cancer patients respond better than others to treatment. After interviewing those who had especially good responses, he found a strikingly similar theme in their answers. All of them had very strong reasons for wanting to live and could elaborate such reasons in great detail. They believed that this strong attachment to a goal in life explained their unusually positive progress. From this, we began to see the importance of building a strong attachment to significant goals in order to develop the cancer patient's inner strength, which is so important in regaining his health.

Often, a patient receiving a diagnosis of cancer begins to restructure his life to live tentatively and conditionally. People begin to withdraw from relationships or refuse to make plans or commitments. This negative expectancy becomes a self-fulfilling prophecy; the patient's mind has been focused on the inevitability of death rather than on recovery. By asking our patients to set goals, usually three-month, six-month and one-year goals, we help them to focus on reasons for living and to re-establish their connection with life. It is a way of reinvesting energy in life by attending to things the person wants and will make an effort to achieve. The will to live is stronger when there is something to live for.

There is some history in the literature indicating that many patients who showed the most dramatic recoveries were those who were physically active as well. Physical activity appears to be an excellent way to relieve stress and tension. Changing one's attention from pains and aches to the exercise itself effectively serves to change the patient's state of mind.

We therefore recommend to our patients a program of physical exercise that we ask all our patients to try. We believe that exercise is another means that the patients may use in participating in their own recovery. We have found that, even for those who are bedridden or who are unable to exert themselves due to pain or other limitations, the visualization of exercise by mental imagery as well as actually moving the fingers, toes, or other parts of the body can support each patient's feeling of doing something for himself.

One of the most difficult phases of working with cancer patients is the strong fear of recurrence of a cancer. When our patients first come to us, we explore their worst fears with them about such a possibility, and we describe what other patients have experienced when they learn their disease has recurred.

Two things become essential for the patients to remember. First, they must reach out to everyone in their support system—

friends, relatives, and the health care team—to be understanding of their mood swings under these conditions. Second, they should not draw any conclusions about what they think the eventual outcome of the disease will be. We ask them to remember that a recurrence may be frightening and painful, but temporary. We also help them to recognize that the recurrence is not a failure but rather that it may have another meaning: Either they may have surrendered unconsciously to the emotional conflicts they face, or they may be trying to make too many changes too fast, which has produced added stress. Still others may have become complacent about changes they initiated and may find it difficult to maintain their changed style of life once the immediate threat of their illness has passed. There are many other possibilities that a competent therapist can help encourage the patient to isolate.

Of course, the most difficult fact of life to face is death. Aside from all of the societal taboos and misconceptions, when our patients are faced with the frightening disease of cancer and all of its implications, it becomes a more immediate, emotion-laden, fearsome prospect for them. The families also find it very difficult to deal with the subject and will even serve to deny such prospects, because they themselves have not come to terms with the prospects of their own deaths.

We have found it essential to encourage the open expression of feelings without judgment. Dr. Elisabeth Kübler-Ross (1970) has observed (and we have seen it in our own experience) that people go through various stages in the process of dying and that some people will frequently not let themselves die, lingering on because a loved one or even a medical team cannot accept their dying. It becomes doubly stressful for them to bear the burden of knowing they are dying and of having to keep up a front for others.

All our work has convinced us that the process of self-regulation in cancer patients is a key psychological factor in the opportunity available to each patient to alter the course of his or her disease. The success they have in helping themselves fight their illness depends upon their belief system and upon how much they are willing to participate actively in helping to change such beliefs.

In summary, we see the psychological processes of illness operating in the development of cancer in the following ways:

1. Experiences in childhood result in decisions to be a certain kind of person. Most of us remember a time in childhood when our parents did something we didn't like, and we made an internal pledge: "When I grow up, I'm never going to be like that." Or we remember a time when some contemporary or adult did something that we regarded highly, and we made an internal pledge to behave in a similar way whenever we could.

Many of these childhood decisions are positive and have an overall beneficial effect on our lives. Many of them, on the other hand, do not. In some cases, these decisions were made as the result of traumatic or painful experiences. If children see their parents engaged in terrible fights, for example, they may make the decision that expressing hostility is bad. Consequently, they set rules for themselves that they must always be good, pleasing, and cheerful, no matter what their real feelings are. The decision that the only way to be loved or to receive approval in the family is to be a certain kind of all-loving person may last a lifetime, even when it makes life a terrible strain.

Some children make an early decision that they are responsible for the feelings of other people and that whenever other people are unhappy or sad around them, it's their responsibility to help them feel better. Possibly, such decisions are the best ones children can make at the time they are made, because the decisions enable them to get through difficult situations. However, in adult life, these decisions of accommodation are probably no longer appropriate, since life circumstances are different from those that existed when the decisions were made.

Our main concern is that the decisions made in childhood limit a person's resources for coping with stresses. By adulthood, most of these childhood decisions are no longer conscious. The same ways of acting have been repeated so many times that awareness of our ever having made a choice is lost.

But unless these choices are changed, they become the rules of the game of our lives. Every need to be met, every problem to be solved must be handled within these limited choices made in early childhood.

Most of us tend to see ourselves as being the way we are just because "that's the way we are." But when the history of our choices is made conscious, new decisions can be made.

2. The individual is rocked by a cluster of stressful life events. Both the research and our own observations of patients indicate that major stresses are often a precursor to cancer. Frequently, clusters of stresses occur within a short period of time. The critical stresses we have identified are those that threaten personal identity. These may include the death of a spouse or loved one, retirement, and the loss of a significant role.

3. These stresses create a problem with which the individual does not know how to deal. It is not just the stresses that create the problem, but the inability to cope with the stresses, given the "rules" about the way he or she has to act and the role he or she has decided upon in early life. When the man who is unable to permit himself close relationships, and who therefore finds meaning primarily in his work, is forced to retire, he cannot cope. The woman whose principal sense of identity is tied up in her husband cannot cope when she finds out that he has been having an affair. The man who learned to express his feelings rarely finds he feels trapped when in a situation that can be improved only if he will express himself openly.

4. The individual sees no way of changing the rules about how he or she must act and so feels trapped and helpless to resolve the problem. Because the unconscious decisions about the "right way" to be form a significant part of their identities, these people may not see that change is possible, or they may even feel that to change significantly is to lose their identities. Most of our patients acknowledge that there was a time prior to the onset of their illness when they felt helpless, unable to solve or to control problems in their lives, and that they found themselves "giving up."

They saw themselves as "victims"—months before the onset of cancer—because they no longer felt capable of altering their lives in ways that would resolve their problems or reduce their stresses. Life happened to them; they did not control it. They were acted upon rather than being actors. The continued stresses were final proof to them that time and further developments would not improve their lots.

5. The individual puts distance between himself or herself and the problem, becoming static, unchanging, rigid. Once there is no hope, then the individual is just "running in place," never expecting to go anywhere. On the surface, he or she may seem to be coping with life, but internally, life seems to hold no further meaning, except in maintaining the conventions. Serious illness or death represents a solution, an exit, or a postponement of the problem.

Although many of our patients remember this thought sequence, others are not consciously aware of it. Most, however, will recall having had feelings of helplessness or hopelessness some months prior to the onset of the disease. This process does not cause cancer; rather, it permits cancer to develop.

It is this giving up on life that plays a role in interfering with the immune system and that may, through changes in hormonal balance, lead to an increase in the production of abnormal cells. Physically, it creates a climate that is right for the development of cancer.

The crucial point to remember is that all of us create the meaning of events in our lives. The individual who assumes the victim stance participates by assigning meanings to life events that prove there is no hope. Each of us chooses—although not always at a conscious level—how he or she is going to react. The intensity of the stress is determined by the meaning we assign to it and by the rules we have established for how we will cope with stress.

In outlining this process, it is not our intention to make anyone feel guilty or frightened—that would only make matters worse. Instead, we hope that if you can see yourself in this psychological process, you will recognize it as a call to action and will make changes in your life. Since emotional states contribute to illness, they can also contribute to health. By acknowledging your own participation in the onset of the disease, you acknowledge your power to participate in regaining your health, and you have also taken the first step toward getting well again.

We have just described the psychological steps we have identified and observed in a patient's becoming ill. It's important to appreciate that many of these steps occur unconsciously, without the patient's awareness that he or she was even participating. The whole purpose of explaining the psychological steps in the spiral toward illness is to build a basis from which the patient can proceed to the steps in a spiral toward recovery.

By becoming aware of the spiral that occurred in the development of their own illness, many of our patients take the first step in altering its direction. Then, by changing attitudes and behavior, they can tip the scales in the direction of health.

We have observed four psychological steps that occur in the upward spiral of recovery:

1. With the diagnosis of a life-threatening illness, the individual gains a new perspective on his or her problems. Many of the rules by which an individual lives suddenly seem petty and insignificant in the face of death. In effect, the threat gives the individual permission to act in ways that did not seem permissible before. Held-in anger and hostility can now be expressed; assertive behavior is now allowed. Illness permits the person to say no.

2. The individual makes a decision to alter behavior, to be a different kind of person. Because the illness often suspends the rules, suddenly there are options. As behaviors change, apparently unresolvable conflicts may show signs of resolution. The individual begins to see that it is within his or her power to solve or to cope with problems. He also discovers that life did not end when old rules were broken and that changes in behavior did not result in the loss of identity. Thus, there is more freedom to act, and there are more resources with which to

live. Depression often lifts when repressed feelings have been released and when increased psychological energy is available.

Based on these new experiences, the individual makes a decision to be a different kind of person; the disease serves as permission to change.

3. Physical processes in the body respond to the feelings of hope and the renewed desire to live, creating a reinforcing cycle with the new mental state. The renewed hope and desire to live initiate physical processes that result in improved health. Since mind, body, and emotions act as a system, changes in the psychological state result in changes in the physical state. This is a continuing cycle, with an improved physical state bringing renewed hope in life and with renewed hope bringing additional physical improvement.

In most cases, this process has its ups and downs. Patients may do very well physically until their renewed physical health brings them face to face with one of their areas of psychological conflict. If one of the conflicts has had to do with a job, for example, the physical disability associated with the illness may have temporarily removed the conflict because the individual was unable to work. With physical health restored, however, the patient may again be facing the stressful life situation. And even with renewed hope and a different perception of self and of the problem, these are usually difficult times. There may be temporary physical setbacks until the patient again feels confident enough to cope with the situation.

4. The recovered patient is "weller than well." Karl Menninger (1959), founder of the Menninger Clinic, describes patients who have recovered from bouts with mental illness as frequently being "healthier than healthy," meaning that the state of emotional health to which they have been restored is in fact superior to what they had considered "well" before their illness. Much the same observation applies to patients who have actively participated in recovery from cancer. They have a psychological strenth, a positive self-concept, and a sense of control over their lives that clearly represent an improved level of psychological development. Many patients who have

been active in their recovery have a positively altered stance toward life. They expect that things will go well, and they are victims no longer.

Although long-term studies have not yet established the success rate of survival, in the limited experience of our own clinic, we find significant instances where people classified as terminally ill or as facing the imminent prospect of death have been able to alter the course of their disease and extend their longevity beyond any medical expectations for survival.

In the past four years, we have treated 159 patients with a diagnosis of medically incurable malignancy. Sixty-three of the patients are alive, with an average survival time of 24.4 months since the diagnosis. Life expectancy for this group, based on national norms, is twelve months.

A matched control population is being developed, and preliminary results indicate that the survival of patients in that group is comparable with national norms and is less than half the survival time of our patients. For the patients in our study who have died, average survival time was 20.3 months.

Many other researchers and clinicians throughout the country are now using variations of the methods we have described, and it is hoped that an accumulation of data will prove to be supportive of these approaches, augmenting the traditional medical therapies now used to treat malignancies.

It has become apparent to many clinicians that the belief system is intimately involved in the catastrophic disorders of cancer. We have seen how changes in beliefs can have an enormous influence on the condition of cancer in some patients.

Children suffer from many of the same fears as adults, but they have their own juvenile world to deal with when confronted with a catastrophic disorder. Dr. Jampolsky has had some remarkable experiences with the clinical use of spiritual psychotherapy, which has benefited afflicted children and their families. Children, like adults, can learn to participate in their own healing process. The power of love as the fuel for healing is demonstrated in this chapter by children learning to help themselves by helping others.

7

Peer Healing and Self-Healing In Children

GERALD G. JAMPOLSKY, M.D.
PATRICIA TAYLOR

The fact that we, as human beings, can learn to self-regulate our internal processes has brought new light on how we can modify our perceptions of both our internal and external worlds.

We are continually increasing our awareness of the limitless power of the mind. Our interest in our self-regulating powers has not been limited to the neurophysiological aspects of body control; on the contrary, the thrust of our interest in the self-regulation process has been in those self-regulatory mechanisms that result in bringing about peace of mind, which can be another way of defining healing.

Peace of mind is clearly an internal matter. It must begin with our own thoughts and then extend outward. It is from our peace of mind that a peaceful perception of the world arises. We all have the power to direct our minds to replace the feelings of depression, anxiety, worry, and fear with those of peace.

This concept has been our major focus in working with children who have cancer and other forms of catastrophic illness. This concept need not be limited; it can have application to both children and adults, regardless of the illness; and it can assist in the maintenance of a positive health profile.

In our concept of self-regulation, the issue of cause and effect is reversed. By this, we would imply that our sense of equanimity and peace does not depend on the conditions of our external environment or on the perceived conditions of our body; our sense of peace is dependent on our internal world and on our decisions to direct our minds to experience peace by experiencing a sense of at-one-ment with everyone and everything.

Putting it more simply, the world and those in it do not cause us pain, and we are capable of training our minds to change all thoughts that hurt. We believe that each of us is responsible for the world he or she sees and for the feelings he or she experiences. It is our thoughts that cause the world we see.

Before going into some of the details of our work, we would like to share with you some personal experiences of one of the authors that tended to stimulate the direction of our work.

INTRODUCTION

It was in 1949 when I (G. G. J.) was interning in Boston that I first became interested in cancer and in something called a "will to live"—and a "will to die." The observation that the will to live can affect the course of an illness is something every doctor really knows in his heart, and yet it can't be put under a microscope, it can't be measured. Yet it is a truth, even though scientists are not able to document it. It became clear to me then that one doesn't have to see something or to measure it for it to be a truth.

Love can meet that same criterion—it is a sense of knowing that defies words—but you can't measure it, you can't see it under a microscope, it has no limits or boundaries, and it is self-creative. Perhaps the best definition of love that I have ever heard is a very simple one: Love is the absence of fear. And love may be the fuel of all healing.

It was also in 1949 during my internship that I became fascinated in learning that, through hypnotic suggestion, one could make a tumorous growth, called a wart, disappear. I began to wonder: Why couldn't you do that with cancer? I then began to do research in hypnosis and began to be intrigued that through suggestion and mental imagery, one can change one's sense of time and space, one can get rid of pain, one can change one's states of consciousness, one can change one's perception and change the illusion of illness. It seemed that there was nothing the mind could not do. The mind did not seem to recognize the word "impossible." I became intrigued at seeing the mind as if it were a motion picture film: All one needed to do was to learn techniques that would wipe the old pictures off so that one would constantly have new blank film; one could create whatever picture one wanted to experience, and then could find that as one's own reality. For the years to come, this became the center of my focus.

When one is attempting healing, it is essential to find a common bond, a joint experience, as a basis of bringing about healing. In 1952, I was head resident of neuropsychiatry at Stanford Lane Hospital in San Francisco. I was called one morning at two A.M. to see a man who had apparently gone berserk in an isolation room on the psychiatric ward. When I arrived at the ward, I found that he had taken the wooden molding from around the door off with his bare hands and was running around the room yelling and screaming, not making any sense, carrying this wooden board with nails sticking out of it. I was supposed to be the person who was to come into the room to help him. There were two orderlies under five feet tall who said to me, "Doc, we're right behind you." I really didn't know what to do. I quickly became aware that I was scared. I was scared that, if I went in that room, I was going to get hurt or that the patient might get hurt, and, after looking into the little window and watching this man, I became aware that he was scared, too. I decided to use this finding, this observation, as a possible bond between us. I yelled in to him, told him who I was and that I wanted to come in there and help him, but that I was really scared that either he or I would get hurt, and that I couldn't help but wonder if he might not be scared too. For the first time, he began to make some sense, and he yelled out, "You're God damn right, I'm scared!" With that, we began to have a conversation with each other, at first yelling back at each other, sharing our fright with each other. As we continued to talk, the fear in both of us became alleviated, and our voices became lower pitched; eventually, he permitted me to come into the room quietly to give him some medication, and he went to sleep. We would like to bring to your attention the observation that, if healing is to take place, it is just as important for the physician or other health personnel to be aware of their own fears and to do something about them as it is to be aware of the other person and his fear. You will be on pretty safe ground when you perceive that other person only as an extension of yourself. Finding a common bond that will heal the separation between you and the person is what is essential.

CHANGES IN WORLD CONSCIOUSNESS

Today, there seems to be a rapidly growing movement of energy that is producing a new awareness and a change of consciousness. It is like a wave of disturbance, a spiritual volcano about to discharge itself on the earth. As we begin to look inward and explore our inner spaces, we begin to recognize the harmony in at-one-ment that has always been there. As one begins to listen to that inner voice, as one begins to surrender to that inner voice, one begins to recognize that true moments of healing and growth occur when all the voices of the physical senses are hushed and silenced, when all personalities have ceased to touch us, and when we have learned to be still. This movement of consciousness seems to be coming from a recognition that the world we see with our physical eyes seems to be destroying itself. Many of us are coming to grips with the recognition that we do not seem to be able to change the world we live in. We do not seem to be able to change other people as much as we would like to, and we don't seem to be able to change ourselves. Perhaps the answer is that we can learn to change the way we look at the world, the way we look at others, and the way we look at ourselves.

Most of us are still going through periods of trying to seek something that we can never find, trying to control and predict. We constantly feel isolated and disconnected, separate, alone, fragmented, unloved, and unlovable. We never seem to get enough, and everything seems to be temporary. Even with those people who are close to us, we seem to have love/hate relationships. Many of us are finding that, even after obtaining all the things one thought one wanted in terms of job, home, family, and money, there still seems to be emptiness inside.

Mother Teresa, from Calcutta, India, calls this phenomenon "spiritual deprivation," and more and more people seem to be becoming aware of this phenomenon. There seems to be a growing recognition of a need to feel a sense of fulfillment within rather than to experience success from without. The results of the stress we perceive in regard to the above are frustrations, depressions, perceptions of pain, illness, and death. Most of us seriously want to get rid of the pain, the illness, and frustrations, but we still want to maintain the self-concept. Perhaps that is why we are going in a circle—because we rigidly want to hold onto our old belief system.

CHANGING OUR BELIEF SYSTEMS

Our belief system is really based on our past experiences, which have resulted from perceptions of the physical senses. In effect, what you believe is what you see. Or, as one comedian put it, "What you sees is what you gets." The belief that our physical senses determine our reality has made man think of himself as a complete and separate entity. It has caused him to see a fragmented world.

The world that we see and that seems so insane is the result of a belief system that doesn't seem to be working. To perceive the world differently, then, means that we need to be willing

to change our belief system, to do away with our misperceptions, to let the past slip away, to expand our sense of nowness,
and to let the fear that our minds have manufactured dissolve.
These are some of the thoughts which led to the establishment
of the Center for Attitudinal Healing.

CENTER FOR ATTITUDINAL HEALING

The Center for Attitudinal Healing, in Tiburon, California,
serves as an adjunct to the medical model for those who wish to
take an active role in their own healing process.

Our model is educational in its format. We work with people
on a horizontal, coworker basis. Everyone is equally interested
in helping to heal him- or herself by helping others. Hence,
everyone is a teacher-student, student-teacher to each other.

The foundation of our work is spiritually based, and we
give our energies in order to bring about a harmonious balance
between spirit, mind, and body. Our emphasis has been to see
ourselves as part of a whole. We have attempted to direct our
goals into experiencing oneness with each other and the universe rather than going in the direction of separation and
fragmentation.

Our definition of healing is to experience peace of mind,
peace of God. We feel that we are all psychotherapists to each
other, in that we are constantly aiming at redetermining what is
real and what is false.

It is our thought that whatever we see with our physical eyes
is only a projection of what is going on inside of us. If our
thoughts are that there is a hostile, attacking world around us,
then that is what we will see. And, conversely, if our thoughts
are that there is only a loving world, then that is all we will see.

Healing, then, has to do with the correcting of our misperceptions.

When the Center for Attitudinal Healing, in Tiburon,
California, was started, *A Course in Miracles* (1975) was the
thought system that formed the matrix of its functioning.

We were interested in establishing a center where people who wanted to take responsibility for their own positive health profile could come. We wanted to create a place not where things were done to them but where techniques could be offered in which they could choose to do for themselves.

Following are some of our basic concepts:

1. Only the mind can be sick—and only the mind is in need of healing.
2. No mind is sick until another mind agrees that the two minds are separate.
3. Healing is the effect of minds that join; sickness comes from minds that separate.
4. Sickness is anger taken out upon the body so that it will suffer pain.
5. No one can suffer if he does not see himself attacked and losing by attack.
6. The errors of belief that anger brings us something we really want and that by justifying anger we protect ourselves must be corrected.
7. In obeying the inner voice, it becomes important to never for a moment be tempted to allow the senses to suggest failure, fear, or doubt.

We make use of meditation, prayer, mental imagery, biofeedback, and other techniques. Much of what we do could be called "spiritual psychotherapy." In using the word "imagery," we prefer the definition that imagination, in its purest sense, is a spiritual ground for the projection of thought.

Contrary to the standard psychiatric theory, we believe that there are only two emotions: love and fear. Love is real and fear is false—something that our minds have manufactured. Since the essence of our being is love, we have everything that we need. The moment we feel that someone else has something we need, sooner or later we will attack that person. At the center, we put our energies in the direction of not putting expectations on others. We practice forgiveness, which we define as letting go and as recognizing that what we thought someone did to us never really occurred.

There are no patients. We are all motivated toward correcting our own errors of perception, which, we feel, results in the healing of relationships. We are all there to be healed and to make alive the statement, "Physician, heal thyself."

What would happen if all the medical personnel and people in the healing professions would see their only function as practicing forgiveness! Perhaps we would all see a lot of healing take place instantaneously. Perhaps we would see the potent force that love has in healing.

At the Center, we attempt to put into practice the following precepts, a process which we think helps us to self-regulate our internal processes.

1. Becoming a love-finder rather than a fault-finder.
2. Giving love rather than seeking it.
3. Seeing everyone as either extending love or asking for help; that is, recognizing that, if we see another person attacking us, we will attack back in some form. So, rather than seeing that other person as attacking, we can choose to perceive the other person as fearful or asking for help. Then it becomes much easier to extend our love.
4. We assist each other in letting go of guilt, of painful memories, and of all the emotional attachments and investments of the past. We attempt to see mistakes as errors to correct rather than things to feel guilty about.
5. We feel that much healing can take place by asking the simple question: Do we want to experience peace of mind, peace of God, or do we want to experience conflict? If we want to experience peace of mind, we will choose to extend our love and to experience the joy that comes from the giving of love that has no boundaries, no limits, no expectations, and no conditions. And if we want to experience conflict, we will want to get something or we will want to evaluate why we are not getting it. Imagine the healing that would take place if, with every communication, we would ask the question: Is this communication loving to the other person and to myself?
6. Finally, we put our energies in the direction of taking a leap of faith to attempt to get out of the dilemma that most of us find ourselves in—feeling angry, guilty, and fearful and experiencing pain and illness—of taking a leap of faith that there is something beyond body and mind and that we are all part of that source. What we see with the physical eyes needs to be replaced by what we know in our hearts—that we are joined and that we are not separate from each other.

The following are some of the basic tenets we had about children before beginning our group process.

1. Children are quite capable of making major decisions for themselves. They need the space and faith that they are capable of making decisions. It has been our experience that healing is enhanced when one recognizes that everyone is our teacher, regardless of age. The following are some newspaper article excerpts that appeared in the *San Francisco Chronicle* on January 26, 1978 (Praul, 1978). They describe a seven-year-old making a decision to turn off the oxygen and to die in peace. Like so many youngsters with cancer, he seems to be a wise old soul in a young body who is instrumental in teaching all those around him.

A precocious seven-year-old Santa Barbara boy, terminally ill with leukemia, ordered his own medical treatment stopped and died, in an unusual case mixing mysticism and personal courage.

Edouard de Moura Castro, son of a Brazilian cabinet minister and a youthful disciple of an ancient Eastern religion, died January 10 after asking his mother to switch off his oxygen machine.

Details of the death came to light yesterday after a volunteer social worker made public the boy's taperecorded comments as he struggled to reach his seventh birthday, describing his thoughts about death and afterlife.

"He said, 'Mother, turn off the oxygen, I don't need it anymore.'" recalled his mother, Barbara de Moura Castro. "I turned it off, then he held my hand and a big smile came to his face and he said, 'It is time.' Then he left."

In his three year battle against leukemia—cancer of the blood forming organs—Edouard—nicknamed Edou and a descendant of Brazilian Emperor Dom Pedro II—lived both at home with his mother and at Cottage Hospital in Santa Barbara, where he received transfusions of 170 pints of blood as doctors tried to forestall his death.

"When you are dead and a spirit in heaven, you don't have all the aches and pains," Edouard told Downey (a volunteer). "And sometimes, if you want to, you can visit this life, but you can't come back into your own life."

Family physician Joseph Delgado treated the seven-year-old as if he were an adult, explaining every treatment and allowing Edouard to make his own decisions.

"Perhaps more youngsters should be allowed to make these decisions in treatments," said Delgado. "Edou knew long ago that he would eventually die." . . .

2. Children can make their own decision of what reality is. They can have an inner sense of knowing that they are at one with everything in their environments. They can also withstand the temptation to be manipulated by their elders to accept the adult standards of what is real.

3. Children, with their fertile imaginations, with their imaginary playmates and their so-called games of make-believe, are experiencing a true reality that we adults may mistakenly call imagination or illusion. Putting it another way, children may be far closer, in our opinion, to knowing and experiencing what is real than the adults around them.

4. Children can learn to control their autonomic nervous systems and their internal processes. Their minds can decide how they want to react to both their internal and external environments. (We have worked with healthy children, aged six to ten years, who are quite capable of modifying their peripheral temperatures and of learning how to relax in a stressful environment, and we feel that this is a way of their taking responsibility for maintaining their own positive health profile.)

5. Children are capable of seeing things as a whole, and they can blend, in a harmonious fashion, spirit, body, and mind, while adults around them are seeing everything and everyone as separate and are fragmenting everything.

6. Children have an innate spiritual awareness that love is the essence of their being.

7. Children are born in innocence and with a sense of oneness and of joining with everyone. They seem to have a built-in knowledge of utilizing prayer as a vehicle for communicating with God.

8. Children seem to be born with a built-in capacity for forgiveness.

9. To the child, reality is not limited to what can be seen with the physical eye. The child's reality is more involved in what he sees with his mind's eye and in the world of what is invisible. What is real to the child is what one doesn't have to experience with the physical senses.

We have much to learn from children. True healing can take place when we allow children to be our teachers. The above factors form the foundation for our group process with children with catastrophic illness.

We might add, parenthetically, that it seems to us that we adults spend a lot of time being seekers in the external world and in outer space, whereas the child is more content to accept his own internal space as all the reality he needs.

At our Center, healing means healing of the mind, dissolving of fear, and experiencing peace of mind in the harmony of body, mind, and spirit. As you can see, categorizations of who the patients and doctors are, of who the healers and healees are, have become irrelevant. We are all coworkers, or brothers, who are interested in healing ourselves.

USE OF IMAGERY IN LEUKEMIA

In the following vignette, we will go into some detail in order to share with you some of the relevance of hypnotic imagery in healing and in the relief of pain, as well as its use in the self-regulating process.

I (G. G. J.) became involved with children who had cancer about fifteen years ago. I had what could be called one of "Maslow's peak experiences" when I was working with a fifteen-year-old boy, whom I will call David, whose pediatrician thought that he was in the terminal phase of leukemia and who was suffering from excruciating pain from both the disease and the drugs. For me, the experience with David seemed like one of those transcendental experiences that I had read about other people sometimes having.

My only contact with David's mother had been a casual one

in social situations. I was also aware that her husband had died of cancer of the lungs two years previously.

One night, when I was having dinner out in Tiburon, California, I noticed her having dinner with a man, and we greeted each other at a distance. Just as I was about to leave the restaurant, she came over to me and stated that her son had leukemia and was in much pain, apparently both from leukemia and from the side effects of the various new drugs that he was taking. Seeing me in the restaurant reminded her that I had a competency in hypnosis, and she wondered if using hypnosis with her son might be helpful. I told her that I had not worked in that kind of specific situation with hypnosis but that, if her physician would want me to work with David, I would be glad to do so.

The situation turned out to be quite complicated. David was confined to his bed and was getting intramuscular shots from his older brother for pain. There was quite a conflict in their relationship. David's mother had developed an alcoholic problem as her way of dealing with all the stress that had come her way. The maternal grandparents were frequently in the home, and their presence seemed to add to the tension. To cap things off, no one had been direct with David about telling him his diagnosis.

On seeing David the first time, I shared with him my lack of experience in this specific area but expressed my willingness to form a dual working relationship with him with the hope that we could learn from each other. It became clear that David really knew of his diagnosis but both suppressed and repressed it in his own effort to protect his family by keeping the "secret."

After I had talked with David's physician, he told David about his diagnosis. This simple interaction did much to relieve the tension, as David no longer had to hide his fear, which, in my opinion, was playing a part in his pain.

David was an excellent hypnotic subject. The method we devised together was a dissociative technique in which he was able to learn to dissociate his mind from his body while in a hypnotic state.

In essence, this meant that he was able to create an illusion whereby he would find his mind separate from his body and could view his body in the bed. He was then able to go one step further and detach himself from the personal pronoun so that he was simply able to see "a body in the bed."

David also became quite competent at using autohypnosis.

David had a strong desire to see the world differently, which, I think, played a part in allowing him to change his belief structure. This factor allowed him to modify his body concept, as well as to develop a sense of timelessness and spacelessness that helped him to detach himself from linear time and geographic space.

Equally impressive was David's ability to utilize the hypnotic process to dissolve his fears, his angers, and his guilt feelings.

Rather than being the "good," "perfect," "uncomplaining" patient, he went through a stage, for the first time, of crying, screaming, and vocalizing his fears and anger. He became aware of the angry feelings that he had toward his father because of his father's dying and deserting him, as well as his angry feelings toward his mother, brother, grandparents, pediatrician, and God, and also toward me.

David was later able to begin to detach himself from some of the emotional trauma of the past and, in a sense, to let go of the past. He would frequently use the imagery of tying these past events to a bird, and he visualized the bird flying away and disappearing. Coinciding with this image, David seemed to be able to begin to forgive others, as well as himself.

These procedures seemed to be quite helpful in relieving him of pain.

I would like now to highlight the three dynamic factors that I feel were mainly in operation during the hypnotic sessions. It is my impression that these factors are relevant regardless of the cause of the pain.

1. Change in the belief system. A change in the belief system takes place that allows the person to look at himself and his inner and outer worlds in a different way.

2. Using hypnotic images to detach oneself from one's body concept.

Here, one uses hypnotic imagery to create an illusion that body and mind are separate. The next step is for the person to allow the illusion to become a true reality for himself. This allows for the concept that the mind controls the body, which is far different from our "awake state," where the body may seem to control the mind. When the body controls the mind, as it frequently does for most of us, it serves to create the illusion that the pain is real and that the disease process is real. The pain seems to serve the purpose, on the one hand, of making the ego feel stronger and more alive, and, on the other hand, of making the ego "muscle-bound" and immobilized. (This is an example of one of the many dichotomies we face as we continue to examine our own behavior.)

3. A change in time conception from linear time, involving past, present, and future, to a concept of timelessness.

One aspect of the hypnotic process that I have always marveled at is the time distortion that can take place.

Pain flourishes when the ego is kept alive by perceiving time as past, present, and future. When one uses hypnotic imagery to go beyond the "alert awake" state of consciousness and to enter another state of consciousness, a most fascinating phenomenon can take place.

As one enters a state of consciousness where there is no time, just a state of timelessness, one's former perception of pain as something real changes to a feeling that pain was an illusion that has disappeared.

Another factor to be considered here is that, when one is dealing with a timeless reality, concepts of "cause" and "effect" disappear. Sequential time, logic, rational sequential thinking, common sense—which seem to be important factors in creating the perception of pain—cease to have a value in this altered state of consciousness.

CHILDREN WITH CATASTROPHIC ILLNESS

At the Center for Attitudinal Healing, when we began to work with children who had catastrophic illness, we found that they had one thing in common—fear.

Dr. Kübler-Ross (1970) talks about the questions adults are faced with when they are told they have cancer: "Why me? Why now?" Children have these same questions but differ from adults because they frequently ask questions nonverbally and express their fears in pictures they draw or in their play.

Children, like adults, when facing the possibility of death, are concerned about separation, isolation, and abandonment. Being in a hospital tends to reinforce these feelings. The night time in a hospital frequently tends to be a particularly devastating time because of their sense of isolation, and it is during this time that these children are most likely to want to talk about what is going on inside of their guts—if only there were someone friendly to talk to who would be nonjudgmental, accepting, loving and, what is more important—nonfearful. Our system frequently does not meet this need. Children do not like to make an appointment for the times when their insides are erupting with the fury of a volcano, so they learn to wear costumes, just as we adults do, in order to disguise their feelings.

Our medical system and hospitals at times get involved in rituals that make it difficult for both the patient and the health personnel to feel human. In these systems, a child may be rewarded for good, conforming behavior and punished for bad behavior. For example, if he or she slows up the system, cries, and makes it difficult for everyone to keep on schedule for x-ray therapy and chemotherapy, the staff may unwittingly reject that child. If he acts like an object and is conforming, he may be rewarded.

In addition, we adults sometimes enter a silent conspiracy with the child not to talk about anything emotional. At times, we may, in a sense, punish the child by saying, "You shouldn't be asking those kinds of questions and thinking that way," and then we change the subject, encouraging the child to suppress those feelings into his inner space.

Children seem to operate as if all minds are connected. They know to whom they can talk and to whom they can't. They have an uncanny ability of getting inside one's unconscious self and of knowing what one is feeling and thinking without any words being said. Once again, we would like to say that children are truly beautiful teachers and that we have a lot to learn from them. All we have to do is create the space for that to happen.

Our culture has a tendency to become fragmented. It has emphasized "separateness" and caused us to split off the body, the mind, and the spirit and to develop specialists that treat each, so we have a minister or priest, a blood doctor, a nurse, a head doctor, and so on.

With the new age consciousness, perhaps we can take a more holistic view and not see a separation of the body, mind, and spirit—either in the other person or in oursleves.

Perhaps we are ready to stop passing the buck to a specialist who is more qualified—be it a minister, a physician, or what-have-you.

Perhaps we can remember that we are all equally qualified to share our love, our total acceptance, and our nonjudgmental attitude with all those we communicate with.

Before going on, let us describe what we call healing and what we think traditional medicine calls healing.

TRADITIONAL MEDICAL MODEL

In medicine, one is concerned with an abnormality of the body. We evaluate, make judgments and comparisons, put parts of people—as well as people—into categories, use measuring sticks, and deduce that a person is ill. We are concerned with what we perceive with our five senses and particularly with what we see with our physical eyes.

We then try to do something to that person that changes his body back to normal—that is, like the majority of people. This is called healing.

Usually, the person is the passive recipient of a treatment on a vertical (an active authority figure treating a passive recipient patient) basis and doesn't take an active part in the healing process. In the traditional medical model, the medical team is interested in healing the "patient" and is not concerned with healing themselves.

In the model we have been using at the Center for Attitudinal Healing, healing can be defined simply as getting rid of fear and bringing about inner peace.

PEER- AND SELF-HEALING GROUP

Our group was formed because it was thought possible—with the children's help—to develop a group process that could meet some needs not yet met by the traditional medical system. The model we have been developing, we believe, could work both inside and outside a hospital environment.

We call this process peer-healing and self-healing. We have long been convinced that children can help each other far more effectively than adults can help children in the healing process.

Children who have cancer or leukemia, or those who face life or death situations, seem to have in common what we mentioned earlier, an emotion called fear.

The inner voice communication of what goes on in these children's minds needs an outlet and an acceptance that frequently is not met. We went to these children and asked for their help to see if we might form a group process that might benefit us, as well as serve as a model for others to duplicate.

The major theme of our group is that, as we learn to heal others, we learn to heal ourselves. In our brand of healing, what is required to bring about inner peace is letting go of fear.

We have found it helpful to create an atmosphere of total acceptance where each of us can feel it is safe to say anything we might want to say. We have put our energies at learning not to make judgments, to overlook the past and forgive, and to see our main functions as extending our love and learning more and more not to attack others.

We have developed a number of active imagination processes that help us emotionally detach ourselves from the past and the future, and we have concentrated our efforts on living more in the nowness of the moment. There has been emphasis on "this instant is the only time there is."

The volunteers and I did some preparation work before we met with the children.

With an effort to detach ourselves more and more from the past and the future, we put our energies in the direction of learning not to use the following words, which keep us attached to the past and the future: limitation, impossible, can't, try, if only, but, however, difficult, ought to, should, words that lead to comparisons, words that categorize, and any words that tend to measure. We would use a mental blackboard and erase these words every time we recognized that we were using them. By beginning to use these words less and less, we found that we were better able to live in a sense of nowness. In a way, one is thereby learning to use the left brain less and less and to de-emphasize the use of logical, sequential, and rational thought processes.

We found this process excellent preparation in using positive, active imagination, and it seems to assist in our beginning to use more of our right brain imagery. It allows one to detach oneself emotionally from the past and future, and it allows one not to get caught up in attempting to control and predict—which is an ego defense and another difference from our traditional medical model.

TAKING OUR MASKS OFF

We have found that, as adults, we often feel attacked by the children we work with in subtle ways, such as when the child isn't progressing. We may secretly believe that the child is making us feel incompetent and guilty. And when we are attacked, we frequently feel defensive and find ourselves unwittingly attacking the child by criticizing him under the guise of being helpful.

We find two approaches helpful here:

1. When we think someone is angry or is attacking us, we choose to see that person not as attacking us but just as being scared.

2. We find that making forgiveness our function becomes a way of emotionally detaching ourselves from the past and of letting our fear disappear.

We also have a belief structure that it is important to learn to take our costumes off and to be mutually open with each other, with the knowledge that we will be mutually accepting of each other.

We have based our work on the beliefs that all minds are joined and that words frequently are not necessary in order to communicate feelings of love and acceptance.

We then went out and made home visits, asking if the children would be willing to help us with a group process—a process which has been mostly self-evolving and not preplanned.

Because the most convenient time to meet for the children was six P.M., it occurred to everyone that we might eat with each other at the Center and then have a group interaction after dinner. The age range has been from seven to seventeen years. We meet twice a month. The focus is on living, not dying.

Everyone in the group—the children, the volunteers—is on a first name basis, and we interact on a horizontal basis (that is, the patient and the doctor are co-equal). We are all interested in healing ourselves of our own fears, as well as in assisting each other. As mentioned earlier, there are no patients: We are there to help ourselves and each other.

GROUP PROCESS

At our first group meeting, in an effort to find a common bond, each of us, the children and the volunteers, shared with each other the things in our lives that we are still most fearful about. As the meeting proceeded and we talked about our fears in an accepting atmosphere, it seemed to us that we noticed that we began to let go of some of them and to feel more peaceful.

Later, we all began to talk about death—our fears about

it, what we imagined it to be like—and we even drew pictures about it.

Simultaneously, the children seemed more free to talk about their innermost feelings at home. They no longer felt that they had to protect their parents from crying by asking too touchy a question. Prayer and meditation frequently became a part of our process.

Almost immediately, we seemed to develop a very strong mutual respect for each other, as well as a respect for the honesty of our communications. We also began to recognize that we were not alone. We were truly teachers to each other, and age was no factor at all.

One example is that of Harry, age seven, whose hair was falling out for the first time. He was scared to go back to school. The older members of the group who had already been through this were extremely helpful to Harry in sharing their experiences and in giving advice.

Then there was Jane, age eleven, who was referred to us because when she was playing at school, a volleyball knocked her wig off. She was completely devastated: She ran inside the classroom, hid under the teacher's desk, and then refused to go back to school. The school nurse had heard of our program, and Jane was referred to us, with the result that we have been mutually helpful to each other.

Many of the children found prayer helpful, and frequently their praying opened up a new spiritual awareness in their families.

One child, John, age twelve, had been quite protective of his parents. He would hide his feelings of fear about his possible death because he didn't want to make his parents cry.

As all the members of the group became more comfortable about talking about their feelings, John began to be more open about his fears and questions at home. In a sense, he became a teacher for his parents, and his parents, in turn, were able to be more open about their feelings with him. When fear vanishes, love flows safely again.

An eighteen-year-old, sophisticated young woman was referred to us with a lymphosarcoma. She wasn't at all sure that she wanted to join a group that had an age span of seven to eighteen years, but she decided to give it a try. She left the first meeting high and excited and amazed that a seven-year-old child could help her with her fear of bone marrow procedures.

This process seems to suggest that, as we lose ourselves by helping others, we seem to develop more strength and confidence at handling the uncertainties that each of us has to handle daily.

USE OF ACTIVE IMAGINATION

We have utilized procedures to assist children in taking an active part in their own self-regulating control of their disease processes. A common denominator in these processes has been making use of active imagination in the form of positive images. For example, many of the children have developed motion pictures in their minds where good cells are winning over the bad cells. This mental imagery allows the child to participate actively in his own healing process. The following pictures are some examples of the children's imagery process (see Figures 7-1 to 7-4).

Henry, age seven, was referred because of cancer of the bone. His best friend had died three months previously from leukemia, and now Henry was going to the same hospital for x-ray and chemotherapy. Henry, as you might imagine, was terrified of any medical procedure and had a tormenting fear of dying.

Henry became involved in our group process, and the other children were extremely helpful to him. He began to use his active imagination and developed mental pictures in his mind of the x-rays and the chemotherapy destroying the cancer cells. He also imagined good fish cells chasing and destroying the bad cells (see Figure 7-3).

As Henry found a way of actively participating in his own treatment rather than just being a passive recipient who was having something done to him, his fear vanished, and he began

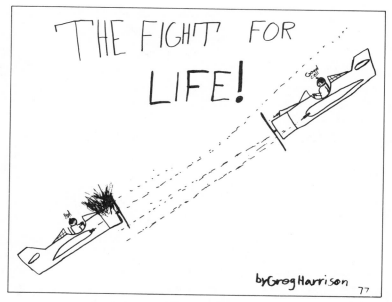

Figure 7.1

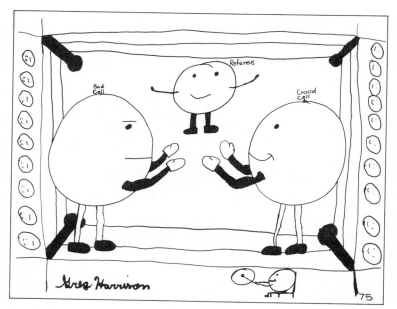

Figure 7.2

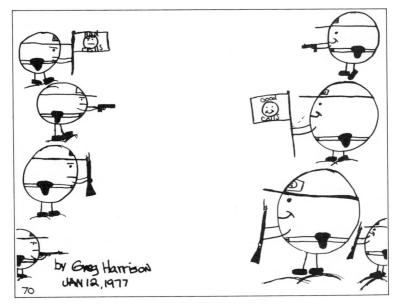

Figure 7.3

Figure 7.4

to cooperate with the medical personnel. Later, Henry was most helpful to new members of our group. Henry really demonstrated that "giving and receiving are one in truth."

A BOOK FOR CHILDREN BY CHILDREN

As the weeks progressed, the idea occurred that we might write a small book for children who are facing a catastrophic illness for the first time—a book for children, written by children, that could be put in doctors' offices, schools, and hospitals. It has now been published and is entitled *There Is a Rainbow Behind Every Dark Cloud* (1978). This book tries to answer questions children have about their own illnesses.

The first part of the book tells about the experiences children in our group had; the second part gives suggestions about the options a child has for participating in his or her own healing process.

We have also started a program in which a child, acting as a peer-healer, and a volunteer visit other children who are just facing the trials and tribulations of a life-threatening illness for the very first time.

OPTIONAL VIEWS OF DEATH

We feel that it is essential to assist the child who has a catastrophic illness, as well as ourselves, to find a harmony between body and mind and to open up options to rediscovering our spiritual selves. Optional models of viewing death as something finite or illusory are discussed in our group meetings at the Center. It gives the child, as well as the health worker, another chance for determining what is real in this world and what is not real.

An eleven-year-old child with leukemia told the group about his feelings about death shortly before he died. "When you die, you just discard your body, which isn't of use anymore, and you go to heaven where you become one with all the souls. Sometimes you come back to earth to act as a guardian angel to someone." He thought that this was what he would do.

OTHER GROUPS

We also have a sibling group which has its own unique problems. Many siblings go through stages where they feel sorry for their brother or sister who has cancer; then they thank God it is not they themselves, which results in guilt. They frequently feel deprived of attention. Later, they may, at times, secretly wish that their sibling would hurry and die so the family could get on with it. Needless to say, we also work with parents. Recently, Children's Oncology Department at the University of California Medical Center in San Francisco asked us to collaborate with them with their adolescents who have cancer.

We are also utilizing the same process with a group of children who have Duchenne's muscular dystrophy. This is a disease that starts about age four years and usually causes death in about eighteen to twenty years.

SUMMARY

We have put our energies into creating an environment where a group process can take place and where one can learn how not to respond in an adaptive manner to an external stressful situation.

Emphasis is placed on the fact that the mind can do anything. As we learn to retrain our minds, we can learn to control our internal environments so that we can have peace of mind, regardless of what the external environment might be.

We stress the fact that the mind can change all thoughts that hurt. Our mind can decide to have peace instead of conflict.

Total nonjudgmental acceptance is the tone of our interaction. We learn that, as we put our energies into extending our love to others and helping others with no expectation of anything in return, we seem to help ourselves.

As we focus on helping others and do away with focusing on our own problems and bodies, fears seem to dissolve, and peace of mind takes their place. Visitors to our group constantly tell us how impressed they were with the feelings of mutual respect, joy, lightheartedness, and love that we all experience. Words fail to adequately describe the experience and the gain received by those who participate in it. Perhaps it can be most simply stated by saying that we all learned that giving and receiving are one in truth.

In terms of longevity, it is not possible for us to state that the interaction that these children had with us played a significant role when there are so many multiple factors, such as chemotherapy, x-ray therapy, and so on, that are happening at the same time. We can say, however, with clarity and conviction, that these children and their families experienced an increase in peace of mind and a diminution of fear.

We have explored what is a consistent fact throughout this book—that man functions in harmony and balance as a natural consequence unless the individual interferes with this homeostasis by faulty thinking or stress-producing thoughts. We have observed how stress can appear in many forms to create all sorts of problems. This stress response comes in many disguised forms, all of which seem to produce the same process—debilitating the individual and impairing his functioning.

In every part of the body, nourishment of cells occurs. These individual cells that compose tissues and organs have an extraordinary system of processing food and other nutrients to feed themselves and to convert whatever nourishment is necessary for the entire body. We have sometimes forgotten that the food for our mind and for our soul is an integral part of the whole person and subject to contaminants that will upset equilibrium, having direct and indirect effects on the physical body. Dr. Goldwag offers a novel approach to the subject of nutrition, recognizing the necessity for feeding the whole man—the body, the mind, and the spirit. The role of self-regulation may become obvious when we realize that we can choose our own mental, physical, or spiritual diets. The decision to choose depends upon our willingness to change the way we view our world.

8

Self-Regulation Through Nutrition

WILLIAM J. GOLDWAG, M.D.

I know just how you feel! One day you decided to take a good look at your health and you said assertively, "I'm going to take more responsibility for the well-being of my self, and the most obvious place to start is with what I eat."

So you got some books and magazines and plunged into the world of nutrition. Chances are that when you came up for air you had a bewildered look on your face. Everyone says something different! In fact, some traditional authorities even state bluntly that the often criticized average American lunch of hamburger, fries, and milk shake provides a reasonably good nutritional content and should be encouraged. Others find fault with the meat, the refined flour in the bun, the saturated fat in the fries, the sugar in the shake, and the preservatives and additives in all three. Who is right? Whom do I believe? Whom do I ask for help? Who really knows? Outside of politics, there are few subjects bound to raise greater controversy and polarity of thought than what constitutes a nourishing diet.

In spite of considerable time and effort devoted to study in this field and to experience in caring for ill people and counseling others, I confess I'm often just as confused as you may be. Remember, however, that one of the side effects of keeping an open mind is experiencing frequent episodes of confusion, particularly when one of your belief systems is challenged. You lose the luxury of holding onto your "facts" when someone else's "facts" seem more plausible. Rather than get bogged down in the nitty-gritty details of the merits of each item of food in the market, it may be of more value to look at the whole field from a larger perspective. Let's first see exactly what we are talking about.

Nutrition is defined as the act or process of nourishing or nurturing. It includes all of the various environmental forces that, combined, act on an organism and further its existence; that is, move it in the direction of aliveness. Notice that there are three key elements in this definition. The first is that there are many and varied forces in the environment acting on the organism. The second is that they act in combination, and the third is that they further its existence and aliveness.

Now you're even more upset! You're trying to simplify things, and I'm suggesting that the study of nutrition has to deal not only with food and its make-up, delivery, purity, and value, but with all the various environmental forces that affect the nurturing of the human in any degree or direction. Even a casual look at the possible number of these astounds us. Whoever first said, "You are what you eat" might better have put it, "You are what you eat, where you eat, with whom you eat, what you see and hear while eating, what you think about or feel while eating, and—oh yes—everything else that ever happens to you!" Certainly, it's a big field, but if we want to know how to nourish ourselves, we have to consider the whole picture.

We must separate out those forces that act destructively, or those that act contrary to existence, from those which aid the life process. Having identified those that are favorable, we must then seek to keep them operating and in close proximity to ourselves in order to encourage the manifestation of their supportive function. Obviously, then, the degree to which an organism's existence is furthered will depend on the balance between these two conflicting processes. At present, it appears that the antilife forces have the upper hand, although it takes them an average of seventy to eighty years to succeed, and, in rare cases, it may take as long as over 100 years. Some progress has been made, since more people make it to that age than in previous years, although there are suggestions that perhaps previous civilizations had some more potent pro-life techniques than we have today that permitted life spans of hundreds of years. In any event, we have much work to do, and I stress this only to dramatize the fact that if we undertake to study nutrition, we must include *all* the elements, not just those related to food.

Now that we have seen how far-reaching this viewpoint of nutrition can be, let us examine some of these varied forces. The obvious ones that come to mind are food, air, and water. Not as obvious are all the other influences that we are exposed to and which enter the body through all the senses. These include everything we see, hear, touch, smell, and taste—and even what we perceive in an extrasensory manner. All these pathways into our bodies provide continuous stimuli, many of which function below the level of conscious awareness, but this in no way diminishes the power of the stimulus to alter body responses. In fact, most of us are aware of only a tiny portion of the stimuli that constantly bombard our sensory systems. Stop at this moment and listen to the variety of sounds going on around you. See how many different ones you can identify. Yet just a moment ago you may have been aware of only one or two. Turn your awareness within and focus on your breathing. Is it regular, deep, or shallow? What sensations can you detect in your toes, your fingers, your bottom, your neck, your jaw muscles? Before you turned your attention to each part of your anatomy, nerve impulses were being fired off from each area. Just because you weren't conscious of them doesn't mean that they weren't in full activity. Every part of your body is constantly sending messages to the brain describing conditions in its immediate vicinity—the temperature, position, amount of muscular contraction, fullness, pressure, tightness, direction, and so on related to the internal environment as well as to the conditions external to the body. All this data is taken in, processed, and assimilated, and it results in what the body considers appropriate response. Thousands of years of evolutionary practice have enabled this remarkable machinery to integrate all these activities and stimuli, ignoring some, rejecting some, and using others to shape and mold the kind of response it deems necessary for the moment. The final step of creation that permits *conscious awareness* of all this activity distinguishes man from the rest of the animal kingdom.

It looks as though we're going to have to examine all the influences that surround us, pick out the ones that are life-sustaining, and assist the people around us to encourage the growth of those beneficial influences while we put no value on the destructive ones, thus minimizing their effect and discouraging their proliferation. This might be considered a great service to our children and to our fellow human beings. Let's begin by considering the large catagory of food.

All animals require living materials in order to support their growth. Most are obtained from the plant kingdom, but many creatures feed on other smaller animals or on those lower on the evolutionary scale. Man appears to have sampled them all, including microorganisms (yeast, cheese, yogurt), fungi (mushrooms), fish, insects, reptiles, and higher animals such as cows, sheep, chickens, and so on. The common factor is that they are all manifestations of life. It would seem wise, therefore, to procure our food with as many of the living ingredients present as possible. In plant sources, this means eating the food as fresh as possible, unspoiled by processing, storing, and preserving, and certainly as free as possible from any harmful additions that may be contributed by soil contaminants and questionable fertilizers, toxic sprays, and other additives. At present, it is a major problem to achieve this state of affairs, since the pressure to produce more crops per acre that are of a uniform color and size and are free from insect damage, as well as the active competition in the food industry for longer shelf life, more varied tastes and textures, and greater convenience in marketing, are all encouraging the proliferation of synthetic foods and newer ways of manipulating the natural product. As a rule, the more processing and altering of the living material, the less nutritional value remains. Particularly unfortunate practices that add much confusion to the unwary shopper are those of refining out many nutrients, of adding back a small number of weaker potency agents than the product had originally, and of labeling the result "enriched." The struggle to obtain greater variety in food seems endless. Perhaps it is symptomatic of man's constantly recurring boredom with what *is* and his constant search for what *could* be.

Good nutrition, then, emphasizes the aliveness of the food and points up the value of yogurts, cheese, yeast, seeds, and sprouts as readily available, fresh, and living biological products. In general, the less cooking, the more nutritional value left in the food. Notable exceptions are products in which the tough outer cellular wall is able to resist the digestive enzymes and requires alteration in order to release the inner ingredients. Soy beans and pinto beans are examples of foods requiring cooking in order to be more healthful. Preservatives added to prolong shelf life in stores, to prevent spoilage, and to preserve original color, may not only turn out to be harmful themselves, but they make it impossible for us to judge the freshness of the food.

The list of additives in food has multiplied to such an extent that we now have as many as 10,000 different ones in use. Their fundamental purpose is to make food appear to be what it is NOT. The kinds of things being used are flavors, both natural and synthetic; flavor enhancers, such as monosodium glutamate (MSG); preservatives and antioxidants (BHT); emulsifiers; stabilizers and thickeners to alter texture; acidulants to change acid-alkaline balance; coloring agents (90 percent of which are synthetic, and many are derived from coal tar); sweeteners; bleaching agents; sequestrants; humectants; anticaking, firming, clarifying, curing, foaming, and anti-foaming products. The urge to do something—anything—to food *except* leave it alone seems to be overpowering. The procedures used to test these additives are notoriously inadequate to provide assurance about safety over the long period that they are in use. That is why the FDA periodically removes some from general use. There is *no* way to predict what effects may turn up after being exposed to some of these chemicals for twenty or thirty years. It is very diffcult to apply what is learned from test animals to humans. Animals are tested under ideal conditions of temperature, health, nutrition, and low stress, conditions which rarely apply to humans, who may also be taking an assortment of drugs that may interact with the additive being studied. Humans are far from homogeneous like animals and are often under great stress, which we know makes all animals more sensitive to chemical assault. One thing is certain: The fewer chemicals you take in, the less chance there is of toxic reactions.

It is likely that the vast quantity of refined, processed foods, particularly those containing large amounts of refined flour and sugar, are responsible for a good deal of the metabolic imbalance in the average adult. Although controlled scientific studies have not shown clear-cut pathology associated with these ingredients, any clinician who questions patients carefully about their diets and behavior patterns will discover a substantial number who have sugar cravings and go on "binges" of ice cream, chocolates, cake, or pie. They will sometimes report brief "highs" after such indulgences, followed by a variety of physical and emotional symptoms including fatigue, irritability, headache, mental fogginess, unclear thinking, inability to concentrate, and so on. Many children manifest marked behavioral changes at home and in school when on high sugar diets. Dr. Ben Feingold (1975) has written extensively about hyperactivity associated with artificial flavors and colors in childrens' diets. Frequently, it is difficult to notice such altered behavior until you switch the child to a more nutritious food plan for several weeks. The contrast in emotional stability may be striking. Sometimes I am amazed at the wide variety of physical ailments that just seem to fade away in some patients when they change from a diet high in sugars and refined carbo-hydrates to a more natural food intake. No one can predict what you may experience; you have to try it yourself.

Another problem with food that is now being more commonly appreciated is that of food allergy. It is only in recent years that we have become more aware of the wide variety of manifestations and symptoms that food allergy may produce. Allergy has become so identified with hives, skin rashes, and respiratory symptoms that we have tended to ignore the many gastrointestinal, emotional, behavioral, and nervous system malfunctions that can occur. The major reason that food allergy has become so prominent is that our diet used to be considerably more varied, but now certain ingredients are exceptionally popular and are found in a great many of the most advertised ready-prepared and convenience foods. Such ingredients as wheat, corn, milk, eggs, and sugars are found in candy, cake, pie, and ready-to-eat food. This frequent repetition of a particular food tends to encourage an allergic tendency to show itself. In addition, radio, TV, newspaper, and magazine advertising is constantly telling us what we *ought* to like and *should* eat. More often than not, it is some kind of highly refined carbohydrate product containing lots of the rapidly absorbed ingredients we mentioned above. This reinforces our conditioning to eat these same foods repeatedly. Elimination diets, sublingual tests, and other methods can reveal these and other unique allergies.

An encouraging countertrend is taking place in some school districts where school lunch programs and vending machines are offering "equal rights" to healthful snacks as an alternative to the plethora of junk foods that, ironically, has proliferated in these "institutions of learning." I suppose the assumption is made that learning takes place only during class hours in certain rooms designated for that purpose. It does illustrate some strange dichotomies to have some economics classes learn about nutrition one hour and to then encourage them to purchase "empty calorie" food because it is profitable to the school cafeteria. It is not profitable to the body's economy. It is in opposition to the life-promoting forces. As mentioned previously, it is not unusual for some health "authorities" to condone the widespread use of many of these "plastic" foods, claiming that numerous people eat them without suffering any apparent harm. It should be noted that it takes years for degenerative diseases to become manifested, and, although more people live to older ages, there is no evidence that their vigor is in any way improved over that of the previous generation. In fact, the nursing home populations are ever-increasing, and we are ending up with larger numbers of nonproductive senile individuals. They are certainly not expressing the life energy.

In summary, then, get your food fresh, live, unprocessed, unaltered, unpreserved, and cooked as little as possible. Eat a variety of food, but eat sparingly of those foods of animal origin. Put more emphasis on a wide variety of fruits, vegetables, seeds, nuts, sprouts, and unrefined grains. Observe the part eating plays in your social and emotional life. It is likely that even the primitive cave dwellers used food as a socializing force; first to form hunting groups (later farming communities) and then to help celebrate feast days. Since modern society has developed so many other social institutions and ways of sharing experiences, there are numerous alternatives to the use of food as "something in common." This would help to curb the obesity epidemic. Experiments suggest that longevity is directly proportional to low body weight.

A discussion of nutritional factors would not be complete without some consideration of food supplements, vitamins, and minerals. Here again, the advocates of these additions to the diet are doing daily battle with the purists, who insist that a good diet provides all the nutrients required. Some of the controversy revolves around a definition of terms. A good diet provides all the nutrients required for whom and for what? If you are referring to the so-called average person (if such a being exists) and are talking about what is required to prevent the well-described classical deficiency diseases, such as scurvy, pellagra, beri-beri, and so on, then diet alone may do it, but what about the fast-growing adolescent on a high sugar diet who is under a great deal of stress at school, sleeps erratically, and goes on crash diets occasionally? Or what about the retired widower who is mildly depressed and lonely and who rarely buys fresh food but subsists largely on TV dinners, canned food, and whatever is soft and mushy because his dentures fit poorly? And what about the borderline deficiency states that don't have a disease named for them because they only vaguely interfere with resistance to other diseases? Their main effect is to reduce energy levels just enough to take the edge off an otherwise zestful enjoyment of daily activities. And let's not forget the traffic policeman in the big city surrounded by smog, car exhaust fumes, cigarette smoke in the precinct lounge, and a bit more alcohol than average when he's off duty. What can we say about the true needs of these people? Add to them the rest of the unusual situations that various individuals present, and you end up with very few getting all their needs from a "good" diet.

Evidence abounds that vitamins C and E have properties that go far beyond their use in preventing colds and strengthening heart action. Many authorities don't recognize these latter benefits, but their lack of toxicity justifies their use in many instances where favorable effects seem evident, even if not provable beyond doubt in double blind studies. Vitamin C may have an even more important role in cancer therapy, along with vitamin A. The potent antioxidant action of vitamin E is highly protective in experimental animals exposed to lethal doses of agents which produce "free radical" reactions. Such reactions can cause premature aging in body tissues.

It has long been known that under the increased stress of prolonged illness or severe infection, certain vitamins of the B-complex family are destroyed at a faster than normal rate. How chronic stress and anxiety may influence this phenomenon is far from clear. The more study we devote to trace elements and minerals, the more we find that there is a great variation in their availability to the body in different areas of the world and even, since climate and land usage fluctuate, in the same area in different generations. An example is zinc, which plays a role in wound healing and is instrumental in restoring taste and smell in some clinical disorders. Supplementation of the normal diet with vitamins, minerals, and other food factors may be very useful and helpful to many people with acute or chronic disease as well as others in satisfactory health who wish to give their body every opportunity to function at its greatest potential level. The difficult question to answer is how much of which ones would be appropriate? Since there is such lack of agreement even among the so-called authorities on these questions, the decisions need to be made inevitably by the consumer himself, using whatever guidelines seem most reasonable to him. To aid him in this process, it is probably wise to do some reading to discover what can reasonably be expected from vitamin use. First, one would wish to know what the general action of each of the major vitamins is, and then one would want to know in what kinds of conditions it has been found useful. It isn't necessary to have absolute proof of effectiveness in each instance, since this is rarely achieved with any drug or medication even after years of study. Each person may not care to wait the several generations it may take to derive such absolute proof. Reasonable approximations are all we have to work with in dealing with the human body.

It is also necessary for the do-it-yourself-er to develop more than a nodding acquaintance with his or her own body physiology. This is not the same thing as a morbid preoccupation with each sensation, searching for some pathological meaning to variations in function. Rather, it is an awareness of recurring characteristic reaction patterns in order to see if there is some common factor such as a food, or even an emotional experience, that relates to a type of body response. The individual is then in a better position to judge whether a particular vitamin or mineral combination is of value. It is, after all, the person's own response to any therapeutic program that really determines how successful that regimen is, regardless of how successful it may be in theory. Inevitably, trial and error is the foundation of all health practice, even if the probabilities all lie in one direction. You may be the exception to the rule.

Water and air are obviously essential elements in our nutritional requirement list. They used to be taken for granted, but today they are becoming rare commodities to find in a pure state. I haven't seen any bottles of air for sale in the market, but when I was a youngster I never imagined I would see drinking water on sale in big cities. Both air and water are suffering from the same onslaught of pollutants which plague our food. The importance of water in the diet has almost been overlooked because of the heavy promotion of soda pop, juices, and flavored drinks. It is unusual for the average child to get a glass of water when thirsty, even though this is generally what his body is lacking. There is a popular belief that milk and juice are better than water. Like so many things in the field of nutrition, one food is *not* necessarily better than another—each may serve a different purpose.

A very common complaint I hear, especially from women, is that of water retention and bloating. This leads to two actions, both of which are very harmful to body dynamics. One is restricting the ingestion of water, and the other is the indiscriminate use of diuretic drugs. Water is retained when there is a temporary mineral imbalance with too much salt in the tissues. The body compensates by holding back water to keep the salt concentration from rising. If you further restrict water intake, there will be still more salt held back, since salt can't be excreted unless there is an adequate flow of water through the kidneys. Similarly, if you force water and salt excretion by diuretics, as soon as you stop the drug, there will be a strong retention. Anyone who has taken diuretics for a while knows how difficult it is to stop them without going through a period of water-logging and, sometimes, frank edema of the feet and ankles.

To counteract this tendency, it is often helpful to actually increase water intake to two or three quarts of water daily. This dilutes out any retained salt and allows the body to excrete extra quantities of fluid. Most of us have lost our sensitivity to water lack and only realize thirst after severe deprivation. After several months of this high fluid diet, you can then let the re-established thirst mechanism guide your needs. It is often advisable to use bottled or filtered water in order to eliminate the unpleasant tastes and dissolved chemicals that are present in many municipal water supplies. Additional problems may be created when certain metals used in the plumbing leach out into the water as it sits still in the pipes during the night, especially where soft water is used and is in the hot water lines. Cadmium can appear from galvanized pipe, and excess copper has been found where copper piping is used. If such conditions exist in your home, it would be wise to not use the first water released in the morning for purposes of drinking or making juice, coffee, or tea. Any contaminants are more likely to be in this water that has been stationary for some hours. As it runs through, the shorter time the water spends in the pipe reduces this effect.

Air is a unique substance in our nutritional portfolio. It contains oxygen, a nutrient that has to be present at all times in order to permit survival. You can go without food for weeks and without water for days, but you can only go a few minutes without oxygen. As a result, air becomes a rather precious ingredient in our daily lives. Yet you would never know it by the way we tend to treat it. Your pet fish get more thoughtful attention to their essential environment, water, than we devote to our vital element. Instead, we pour all manner of dirt into it, such as carbon monoxide, sulfur dioxide, tobacco smoke, auto exhaust gases, and a multitude of particles like asbestos, lead, and others—to say nothing of many radioactive by-products of nuclear reactions. If you like statistics, in 1968, approximately 195,000 tons of lead was discharged into the air throughout the United States, most of it coming from auto engine fumes. Lead serves no useful function in the body and is not easily excreted. Published data which gives "safe levels" of lead in the body are based on the amounts known to cause recognizable damage to the body. But what about unrecognized damage? It is well known that safe levels are arbitrary figures, selected by a consensus of workers in the field and subject to revision as new data comes in. That data is generally the end result of someone's personal tragedy. The experiences with vinyl chloride and asbestos, which were once thought safe to inhale and are now, twenty to thirty years later, realized to be potent carcinogens, are sad reminders that very few foreign substances in the air are absolutely safe.

Now let us turn to the less obvious sources of our nutrition: sensations from inside and outside the body that are perceived by the sense organs. The importance of external sensations in nourishing the human is underscored by the observation that infants not held, fondled, or spoken to will fail to thrive and may die. Sensory deprivation is as traumatic to the nervous system as failure to receive adequate food and water is to the rest of the body. Prisoners subjected to solitary confinement for long periods report a feeling of great relief even to prolonged, painful questioning by their captors. Any kind of human contact is preferable to total isolation. Total sensory deprivation is impossible to achieve, since gravity exerts a force on the body, and, even in a floating state suspended in water, there is pressure on the skin. Even under such conditions, awareness of inner sensations is present. Under experimental conditions, sensory lack will result in a variety of hallucinatory experiences, both visual and auditory. It seems as though the human creates his own sensations if none are provided. It is well known that if vision is suppressed in one eye by a refractive error or eye muscle weakness in childhood, the retina will not develop and permanent loss of vision can occur. Muscles not used will atrophy. Bones not subjected to stress or movement will decalcify. It was stated earlier that all living things consist of movement in some form. Lack of movement is death. Anyone dealing with older people knows this very well. Allow them to stop moving any part of the body or using any function, and it dies. Good nutrition means fostering movement.

Light is another basic prerequisite for life. Sunlight makes plant life possible, and the energy stored by the plant as well as the oxygen released in the process permit the existence of the animal kingdom. Light organized in patterns allows the retina of the eye to define form; we call this process vision. The nature of the light as well as the forms outlined can be nurturing or not, depending on the wavelengths of the energy and the inter-pretation of the forms. We have yet much to learn about how flowers bloom, about how animals reproduce, and about how humans respond, depending on night and day cycles and on wavelengths of light. Dr. John Ott (1973) has done a great deal of pioneering work on the characteristics of light and its effects on living systems. He has found that fluorescent light can cause headaches and even changes in menstrual cycles. Full spectrum lighting is now used to encourage plant growth, and in newborn nurseries it is effective in treating jaundice in newborns. Light-ing creates moods. Sometimes the effects are highly disruptive to the nervous system. The flickering strobe effect in disco-theques creates unusual sensations in the dancers, sought after for their novelty, but disturbing to physiological harmony. In sensitive persons, convulsive seizures can be precipitated by such a visual onslaught. The lower instincts of man are very adept at employing the negative effects of sensory stimuli, and although I dislike referring to the destructive use of various sensations, they can teach us something about the response of the body to various vibrational frequencies. Brainwashing methods employ bright lights to fatigue and disrupt normal neurological pathways in order to prepare the victim for the input selected. Contrast this with the soft lights and music employed by the lothario to create a romantic setting for his planned conquest.

Even subtle variations of light in the form of color are recognized as having distinct properties that contribute to the total nutritional picture. There are pleasant colors, exciting colors, depressing colors, sensuous colors, healing colors, and all the variants in between. Many of these are based on conditioned responses by the receivers, but some may reflect color fre-quencies selected by nature for specific purposes. It certainly appears to be more than just coincidence that the plant king-dom is predominantly some shade of green. The food industry is very mindful of the effect of color on appetite and does not hesitate to make apples more red or lemons more yellow if it sells more of the product (which it seems to do).

Seventy-five to eighty percent of our sensory input is visual. These impressions in infants and children largely determine their conditioning. Among the first visual contacts the infant makes are the eyes of the mother. One could spend hours arguing which is more important, the breast or bottle and its contents or the nature of the eye contact with the mother. The infant reads the whole story of its role in the family in the eyes it sees. Love, resentment, boredom, hostility, anger, preoccupation, threat, daydreaming—all these may be registered here, and each will color, to a degree, the relationships the child will later establish. Those eyes will either help him grow and develop a fuller potential, or they will erect obstacles and tensions that will force the child to erect defenses of his own to deal with what he imagines is there (or not there). From then on, his eyes will bring an incredible variety of images, all of which will be shaped and molded by what his conditioning tells him it's all about. The stronger his conditioning, the more restricted will his vision be, seeing only what he has learned to expect and overlooking or rejecting what is unexpected. Further values, also derived from his conditioning, will be put on what he sees, and the world will then become either an enjoyable, satisfying place where he can grow and attain limitless understanding or a hostile enemy that has to be fought and conquered and that never seems to give him the "more," "better," and "different" that he continually seeks. The former "nutrients" will contribute to his aliveness, the latter to his destruction. What he chooses to see about him, read, or watch on TV or in movies will reinforce either his positive or negative viewpoint. If positive, he will accept what he sees as what *is*; if negative, he will be a victim of every form of manipulation of which society is capable.

Sound is perhaps the second most potent "nutrient" in the sensory system of perception. Like light vibrations, sound vibrations have a whole spectrum of effects on the living organism, and each characteristic of the sound, such as loudness, pitch, and timbre, has its own range of influences. Combining these variations in characteristic ways creates music, and this too has a wide variety of repercussions on living structures. Some types of music are soothing and highly nutritious to life; others tend to disintegrate and disorganize sensitive beings. You might contrast the relative age of performers and conductors of classical music (who enjoy greater longevity) with that of musicians producing the harsher, louder, more abrasive music represented by hard rock. The rhythm also affects the musculature, and kinesiologists now claim that the accented last beat of three-quarter time, common in rock music, produces a weakening effect on muscles, while the accented first beat, as in waltz tempo, strengthens the same muscles. The soothing effects of certain sound combinations are used in dental practice, operating rooms, and doctor's offices to aid in mobilizing healing effects.

Any loud noise is poor nutrition for the infant. He is nurtured by a soft, singing type of voice, which very soon is associated with pleasant feelings of being held, given food, and kept dry and warm. Later, minute changes in inflection in the sound of those voices tell him that he is OK or not OK, that he has performed well or not, or that something is disturbing the source of the sound. In his innocence, he may think the disturbance is his fault, since it is directed toward him. He receives more communication from the quality of the voices coming at him and from the associated facial and body movements he sees and the muscle tensions he feels in the arms that hold him than he does from the actual words spoken. That is why "I love you" is a transmitted feeling and is almost meaningless as a phrase. He senses "I love you" or "I don't like you" long before he knows what the words mean. If he frequently senses "I don't like you" but hears the words "I love you," a confusion and conflict between words and feelings is created and may be carried with him through his entire life, making it impossible for him to correctly identify and interpret loving words or feelings from another person. Quality of voices and intonation will always convey feelings of security or insecurity, relaxation or tension, pleasure or pain, and so on based on these early impressions, and he will choose his politics, spouse, clothes, and health by the re-creation of the sights and sounds that accompanied his emerging feelings.

Sensations from the environment impinge on the surface of the skin and stimulate specialized nerve endings. They, in turn, transmit impulses to the spinal cord, to the lower brain centers, and, in some cases, to the higher brain centers, where they are interpreted as hot or cold, as painful, as light touch, or as deep pressure. Fortunately, most of these sensations never reach conscious awareness or else we would be so deluged by the barrage of impulses that there would be little time to devote to anything else. Add to these external stimuli the millions of bits of data provided by the sensations received from the muscles, joints, and tendons, letting us know the position of every part of the body, and from the inner organs, letting us know about hunger, thirst, fatigue, or the need to empty the bladder or bowels, and you get a hint of the tremendous amount of information being processed from the sense of touch. This contact with ourselves and our environment also has positive and negative nutritional value. We learn to suppress much of this reporting mechanism and, in this way, lose contact with a lot of the messages being sent by our bodies informing us of what is going on. Then we appoint specialists, like doctors, to try to interpret the messages for us. At best, the doctor's interpretation is merely a secondhand image of what only we can experience in ourselves. He puts a name on our experience and calls it a "symptom" or a "diagnosis," but that does nothing to relate what is going on. If we are to derive any benefit from knowing what is taking place, we need to tune in to various parts of our body and to relearn what it tells us about its functional state.

We see, then, that by ignoring the signals sent from inside or from the skin, we deprive ourselves of a rich source of information about the welfare of our inner structures and how to keep them in a better state of balance. Most of us have lost all ability to determine accurately how much food we actually need and what our system is lacking. Instead, we rely on a restaurant or hostess or even a spouse to make the decisions about how much we should eat or about what type of food is best. We even eat when the stomach says "enough," especially if the icing is appealing or the whipped cream beckons—or if the kids were a hassle today or the house is messy or things just didn't go right at the office. Think of how much energy is lost in the unnecessary tension of the muscles or in the inefficient movements of our body that we learned and that we continue to perform out of habit. Often, we have learned in infancy to lock certain muscles and joints in rigid position as a protective device against what we perceived as a threatening environment. This "muscular armor," as it was referred to by Wilhelm Reich (Lowen, 1975), continues to restrict movement and create muscle spasms throughout life, but the original survival intent is forgotten, and the sense of tightness is no longer consciously perceived. This continued contracted area affects function in that region and throws off balance in neighboring areas of the body. Eventually, enough disturbance can result to create pathology of various types. Of course, during this time, some of the original emotions associated with the "armoring" are also locked up, and not only does the physical body's movement suffer, but there is less freedom to experience full emotional activity.

Movement therapies such as bioenergetics, Reichian therapy, and Rolfing concentrate on releasing the blocked energy by physically stretching and manipulating the tissues, thus freeing the emotional content as well as the muscular tightness that guarded it. This opens up the individual to a wider range of environmental nutrients, such as love, affection, compassion, and understanding, not previously available.

Exercise not only feels good to the body, but it is a nutritive procedure. Every time muscle fibers contract, they release potassium from the interior of the cell into the tissue fluid spaces and eventually into the blood stream. Potassium, when available in this form to the heart muscle cells, enables them to utilize oxygen more efficiently, thus reducing the demands for additional blood flow through the coronary arteries. Contraction of muscles anywhere in the body exerts a squeezing action on all the surrounding tissues. This aids in moving tissue fluids and expedites the transfer of nutrients into the cells and of waste products out of them. In the legs, this muscular pumping action helps propel blood through the veins, aiding return of blood to the heart. Other dynamic effects on cardiovascular fitness have been repeatedly demonstrated and written about. There is almost no disability so great that some type of exercise cannot be applied to some part of the body. The results are sometimes astounding. It almost seems as though the life principle gets pumped back into areas other than the parts being worked on. As more people rediscover walking, jogging, and hiking, more attention will be directed to the air quality, the preservation of open space, and the conservation of resources so that the entire ecosystem can benefit.

Another aspect of touch is its potential value as a healing technique. In this respect, it shares with sight and sound a pathway into the body from outside stimuli or from other people. The sight of certain colors, or of a smiling face, the combination of certain tones or melodic sounds, and the warm touch of a friendly hand, pressure on certain sensitive points on the surface of the body, or the massage of certain deeper structures have the power to evoke a healing response from within the body. This response is still not totally clear or definable, but it certainly is there and is put to good use by the wise or experienced physician. This powerful energy system has been largely ignored by Western medicine in its zeal to employ more and more sophisticated drugs and surgical techniques in the treatment of disease. Fortunately, in recent years, the art of healing has again become of interest to therapists, possibly because the list of available drugs is getting so long that it precludes intelligent knowledge of their uses, side effects, and toxicity by the individual practitioner. Here again, the nutritive value of another's touch may overshadow the benefits obtained from food or medicine. The technical cultures have tended to minimize the physical contact between people and have reduced the interpersonal nurturing that can occur when people are allowed to come into close touch with each other. Many of the psychological therapies today emphasize touching as a way of restoring this additional means of support and communication.

As people share experiences and express compassion through physical contact, there seems to be not only an outflow of energy from each person but also an enhanced receiving of loving feeling. Unlike material things, what you give away in love and compassion returns in multiplied degrees as a powerful nutritive force. There are many who have found that the same principle applies even to material goods.

The senses of taste and smell are not developed to the same degree in humans as in animals, probably to some extent because we have placed less importance on them and also because of evolutionary trends. The usefulness of odor and taste are largely confined to evaluation of food now, but there is great advantage in being able to smell (smoke for example) and taste (poisonous substances) accurately. We have helped pervert these senses by our emphasis on gross taste rather than on subtle flavors. The taste buds are so overwhelmed by the need to have everything taste sweet that the threat to remove the artificial sweetener saccharine from the market by the FDA resulted in an indignant outcry from a population who must have their sweet taste at any cost. Once we stop adding sweetness to foods, we discover a variety of flavors we hardly even suspected existed. Developing finer, more highly sensitive taste and smell appreciation is growth; blunting these senses by overwhelming them or by reducing their finer discriminatory powers is against the life principle. Unfortunately, these two senses are used as targets for the food industry to get us to eat more "junk" foods, thus diminishing the aliveness factor. It is a subversion of the normal protective function of these two sensory functions.

So far, as we expand our definition of nutrition, we have touched upon some of the environmental forces that act upon the organism. A key word in the definition is that these forces act in *combination* to further the existence of the organism. This brings us into some conflict with a major technique of the scientific world—the "controlled study." The purpose of this procedure is to determine how responsible a particular drug, manipulation, or factor is for a given effect by excluding all other possibly active materials or factors from a study group and by using another comparable group that is not given the factor under investigation. Such a technique is considered more accurate if you can eliminate all but one variable. To make it even more refined, it is customary to "double-blind" the study, so that the participants don't know which group is the control and which is receiving the active factor; even the experimentors are unaware of who the test subjects are or of what they are receiving. It is generally accepted that this scheme eliminates conflicting influences on the problem being studied and minimizes bias on the part of enthusiastic investigators from affecting the results. This makes good theory and works well in pure research. Unfortunately, Nature doesn't operate in this fashion. Natural phenomena stress the interrelationship of things and events, their interdependence and interaction, not their isolated performance. By ignoring Nature's principles, we are tempted to apply animal study data to humans and to equate performance of one human or group of humans to another. We tend, then, to ignore the fact that all conditions are in a constant state of change; as meticulously as we try to reproduce conditions in test groups, the variable factor of change sneaks in and confounds the results. Perhaps this is why even science finds its dogmas and "certainties" being upset every so often by a new "belief." Phenomena occur because of an infinite number of events preceding (and perhaps even following) them, and the attempt to isolate one or several events and label them as "causes" is a prelude to eventual disillusionment and frustration.

It is this "combination" of factors and their interrelationship that inspires evolution by selecting the factors most favorable to the organism and by encouraging their repetition. It is true that this makes it very difficult to study reactions in humans to any variation in diet, climate, or drugs or to social, psychological, or physiological process. We can develop certain hypotheses based on controlled studies, but when we allow them to solidify into dogma or assume that phenomena occur naturally in the same fashion as we study them, then we violate Natural Law. The true definition of nutrition accounts for this fundamental concept by including the phrase "in combination" to stress the fundamental interplay of all influences in living structures. Nature's key words are harmony and balance. They presuppose a multiplicity of active forces. These forces must act harmoniously for them to be nutritive or life-sustaining. For example, an animal cannot be in a state of alarm and at the same time experience hunger and have the digestive enzymes secreted. Each of these functions alone is beneficial to life and supports the animal's growth, but if they occurred in combination, they would result either in the animal being unable to defend itself adequately or in impairing its ability to break down food and absorb it properly. Nature has set up the controls in such a manner that each of these functions operates at the proper time and under the proper circumstances to accomplish the overall nurturing of the animal. If you studied each of these systems separately and in isolation, you would fail to appreciate how the alarm reaction not only triggers the necessary chemical and neurological sequences to prepare the body for "fight or flight" but also inhibits the digestive and reproductive systems, which are not needed at that moment.

This unfortunate tendency to isolate functions in order to study them without their normal influences has led to a fragmentation of the picture of how higher animals operate. In the field of medical practice, this has resulted in treatment of organs and disease (i.e. "liver", "heart", and "diabetes" or "arthritis" specialists) rather than people. We now speak of "holistic" medicine—that is, treatment of the person as a whole unit—as though it is a new concept, when in reality it has always been the foundation of understanding the complete organism that has become overshadowed by the temptation to separate the elements of the "combination of forces" that comprise nutrition. Perhaps one reason for this tendency is the ease with which the scientist can study elements in isolation. The psychologist Abraham Maslow (1970), referred to this as *means-*centering; that is, the practice of considering that the essence of science lies in its instruments, techniques, procedures, and methods rather than in its problems, questions, functions or goals. Such stress on technique plays down the vitality and significance of the problem and of creativeness in general. If the method is okay, the project is applauded; if it is faulty, it is criticized to death, although the concept uncovered may be of great importance. Even triviality becomes endowed with prestige and status if the method is satisfactory. This is borne out by the multitude of scientific journals and publications with innumerable articles on every conceivable subject. Means-centered scientists, then, fit their problems to their techniques and may even avoid asking or considering certain questions if the currently available techniques are inadequate to answer them. Such people are unable to exist comfortably in the midst of the unknown, the apparently chaotic, and the mysterious. Yet this is where harmonious combinations take place in nature, inexorably pursuing the path toward growth and nurturing, but collapsing like a marionette whose strings have been cut when one tries to isolate each essential factor and sever its vital connection with every other neighboring force. Means-centering also creates a scientific orthodoxy that tends to block the development of new techniques if the method turns out to be too unorthodox. Science professes to search for truth, insight, and understanding and is concerned with important questions. The artist, poet, and philosopher are also vitally interested in these areas; *problem*-centering makes them all collaborators. Such an approach is essential in dealing with the complex interplay of forces affecting the living human.

Another few words must be devoted to "balance." We use the word freely, implying that it is an ideal state, one we need to strive to achieve; however, it is important to realize that balance is conformity with Natural Law. It is the only state that is tolerable in Nature. We need not put out the least effort for it. It operates whether we are aware of it or not and especially whether we like it or not. Imbalance is corrected immediately by Nature by any of an infinite series of responses designed to maintain equilibrium. All of our accepted laws and principles of physics exist with the understanding that events influence each other. Action equals reaction. Matter cannot be destroyed, only transformed. Energy put in equals energy gotten out. Equations mean that one side *equals* the other side. Balance. Unstable states exist only briefly until compensating forces are expressed in response. Step off a cliff and you remain *unbalanced* in mid-air for an infinitesimally short interval. Gravity overcomes inertia and air resistance, and balance is restored as you fall through space. No effort is required on your part to restore balance.

Let us use this understanding to visualize some physiological processes in the human body. There is technically no such thing as a state of *imbalance* in the body chemistry or physiology. Each change in these systems is accompanied by a compensating response. This is called adaptation. Contract a lot of muscles, and more blood flows to them. The heart beats faster; as oxygen is consumed, breathing speeds up and gets deeper. It's all automatic. If your body gets invaded by certain viruses or bacteria and your defenses lag, body temperature rises, and certain areas start to hurt. The body is adapting. You don't like the way it feels? Who said you had to like adaptation? You might not like falling from the cliff, but if you create those conditions, balance expresses itself—like it or not.

What we call disease, then, is merely a series of adaptations (otherwise called signs and symptoms) mobilized by a fantastically complex system that keeps adjusting itself in order to try to preserve its survival. Rather than view the manifestations of the illness, perhaps we could create a new set of circumstances more like those prevailing when there was no necessity to adapt in the manner chosen by the body. One thing is clear. It seems fruitless to try to force your body to compensate in a totally different way than it has done all your life and that thousands of years of evolution have programmed your genes for. Why not reinforce the proven healing capabilities that have also evolved and thus encourage true healing instead of symptom alleviation?

The third important factor in our definition of nutrition is that the varied combination of forces acts in the direction of aliveness. This is not as simple to appreciate as it may seem. Aliveness is not the same as comfortable, nondisturbed, or unperturbed. On the contrary, aliveness requires movement and change, not stasis. As we evaluate more carefully some of our trends in society, they may seem to be attempts to make life easier and less of a strain and so preserve energies for a longer, happier life. This undoubtedly was the concept behind mandatory retirement at age sixty-five. However, it was forgotten that a happy life requires living—which is movement and activity. The ultimate results of stagnation, loss of a place in society, and mental deterioration don't result in a happy, long life but rather in premature senility and death. We have gotten the notion that if only we had more, better, and different jobs, money, or spouses—you name it!—we would have it made and would therefore live happier ever after. This struggle to accumulate and achieve is not nurturing, since it more often leads to discontent, frustration, disappointment, illness, and premature death. Constant awareness of what we are and what we are doing and of seeing where we put value is a potent aid in applying the nurturing energies in the proper direction.

Really seeing where we put value requires some practice. If someone asked you what you value, you would probably answer with several items that you have been told throughout your life you're *supposed* to value. They are what our authorities say we should value. But how do we separate what we actually value from what we think we *ought* to value? There are some easy ways to tell. First, what gets our time and energy? What we actually do most of the time is where we place value. We may offer justifications and reasons for why we *have* to do this or that, but the fact remains that we occupy our time with what we regard as valuable. What thoughts are we occupied with? This is where we are. You may say, "Well, so-and-so has this illness which takes her time and energy. Do you mean she wants to be sick?"

She may not consciously *want* to be ill, but if she invests a lot of time, talk, thought, and behavior in it, it can only be that it is of that much value to her to do that. Others, despite handicaps and illness, put little value on it and so end up involved to a lesser degree in the illness. Where is the time spent? That's where the value is. It may not be what the person admits to or is even aware of, but we cannot invest time and energy in any other way. A useful exercise is for each of us to list what we think we value and then list where our energy and times goes and see how alike (or different) the two lists are. Seeing clearly will enable us to match the two lists more closely.

Seeing this, then, gives us the choice of placing value elsewhere if we wish. This gives us a degree of freedom in our lives that is a step toward aliveness. Good nutrition is placing value consciously where we choose. Conversely, poor nutrition is being at the mercy of everything around and allowing our conditioning as well as our authorities to decide for us what is of value and then carrying out their wishes mechanically.

When we behave mechanically, like machines, then we must expect the deterioration that goes with machinery—rust, wear and tear, falling apart. Acting like a living being brings into play self-repair, self-healing, and regeneration. This separates the living from the nonliving. Man seems to be the only species that has the possibility of choosing which way he can go. Most of us choose to go the familiar, comfortable, easy route that we are taught to expect. Others select the more difficult way of renouncing the past and the conditioning, of not being concerned with the unknown future, and of staying 100 per cent in the present. This is what nourishes the spirit and ultimately constitutes the aliveness of the person. Some are more "alive" than others. Some may even be eternal.

Invariably, when any attention is devoted to the evaluation of non-traditional methods of treatment through history, one is always led to study the remarkable success enjoyed by shamans, medicine men, and other members of a particular culture's health care team. There are many phrases and explanations used to describe this phenomenon and whence it came. When the dust settles, one can find some evidence of a belief in some supernatural force most often thought of as a spiritual aspect of a person's belief system.

In modern society, we have learned to apply many sophisticated sounding phrases and technical words to explain this force in language more acceptable to a scientifically oriented society. But, always, we get back to the same thing. We seem to avoid the direct confrontation with our own feelings about a Supreme Being, perhaps because that Being is often characterized as some gray-haired, bearded figure, looking much like a man, but sitting on His throne in judgment of us all. When one can remove this stereotype from consciousness and be comfortable with the concept of a force or energy that permeates all living matter and is the essence of the Universe—an order, a plan, a rhythm—it becomes easier to recognize the metaphysical basis for a spiritual understanding of our concept of God. Dr. Marcus Bach is an extraordinary observer of the spiritual phenomena of life, both through his studies and in his experiences with human beings throughout the world. He finds the common denominator that connects various systems of thought related to living "whole" and making available those spiritual powers that affect our health and well-being. We always have the choice of exercising what is available to us for better regulation of our lives.

9

Spiritual Power
In Holistic Healing

MARCUS BACH, PH.D.

With the coming of holistic medicine, a new perspective is focused on the effectiveness of spiritual power in today's health care field. Medical science wants to know what religion knows about the subject, and dedicated leaders in religion are just as anxious to learn how much of their knowledge will be confirmed by scientific standards of objectivity.

Such collaborative research has been long overdue. What *is* spiritual power? What are its vital components? Is it something reserved only for "believers?" Is it merely a convenient term to describe the healing force of nature? How does it work?

Religion, always an expression of the attempt of the human psyche to achieve a sense of direction and security in the world, now finds itself in the exciting role of catalyst, an integrating agent in a project involving life's universal triad: body-mind-spirit. Holism presents this invitation to catalytic cooperation not only to religion and to scientific communities but to all seekers for truth who have long been aware of the close relationship between states of consciousness and states of health.

The history of religion indicates that a firm belief in spiritual power is an adjunct to health and healing. Our contemporary scene, rich in its enthusiasm for dynamic living and fitness for life, is prepared for both a re-study and a deeper exploration of the subject. Despite the theological differences and sectarian dissimilarities that still separate various faiths, a common bond of understanding has always been and continues to be the belief that there *is* a special, secret source of healing issuing from a "divine dimension" beyond the limitations of the physical realm.

It is the prospect of discovering and more fully utilizing this wellspring of power that constitutes the present challenge. Here is an exploit as fascinating as the search for the headwaters of the Nile. And, as in the case of the Nile, where the power of its flow was better understood when its long-hidden source was made clear, so this united holistic endeavor for deeper insight into the "river of spirit" has all of the elements of high adventure as well as the added incentive of new discoveries that could contribute to the health of both the individual and the society at large.

What is spiritual power? It is a term related to belief in a supernormal energy which, to the believer, becomes an innate, normal function of being. It is a mysterious force not fully explainable, creating phenomena in and among people of all religious persuasions, which is to say that no one institutionalized faith has a corner on it and that many sincerely doubt that it can be institutionalized. A highly respected researcher of the subject, Manly P. Hall (1977), has concluded that "the art of healing was originally one of the secret sciences of the priestcraft, and the mystery of its source is obscured by the same veil that hides the genesis of all religious belief."

As in the case of acupuncture, where there is no confirmed evidence either as to how or when the meridian system was discovered or to how the cures by acupuncture are effected, so the secret power of spiritual healing is cradled in the predawn of history.

Many persistent archaeologists and other scholars have explored the past and unfurled the ancient scrolls, but what they found in their investigations was rarely palatable to the preconditioned tastes of medical scientists or theologians of the established church. After all, these "primitive" religions, as they were often called, had the audacity to personify their gods and to associate their deities with certain maladies, suggesting an all too polytheistic approach. There was Genetyllis, goddess of childbirth; Hygeia, watcher over sanitary practices; Panacea, symbol of curative powers; Ophthalmitis, queen mother of eyesight; and numerous other *numen* and messengers of healing whose names nonetheless did find their way into the history of medicine. Somehow, their critics failed to see that these personifications were focal attributes by which the patient could visualize a divine helper for his or her particular distress and could find someone to turn to, someone who cared.

Journeys to specific temples in order to receive the healing gifts of the gods, especially to the *abatons* of the famed Greek, Hippocrates, at Kos, held special spiritual power for determined devotees and not only effected cures but helped to shape their dreams. But, again, treating the spirit for physical malaise or adjusting the patient's mind for release of bodily anguish did not seem feasible to sectarian censors of ancient faiths, and we are only now, in the light of new and deeper esoteric understanding, discovering truths that were ignored during moments of righteous indignation.

With the coming of holism comes a renaissance of empathic insight bridging the years and drawing religion and science closer together. Such a partnership is inevitable inasmuch as spiritual power itself is dependent upon the art of seeing the unseen and upon developing a greater openmindedness for investigative research. For although there are still many speculations as to how spiritual power "works," that it *is* connected somehow with the invisible nature of life can no longer be disregarded, and an awareness of the fact will help us in our quest.

Awareness is certainly one threshold at the door of holism's entrance into the life of our time. As physical theories of disease have decreased and the importance of the integration of body-mind-spirit has become more compelling, as the emotions, the psyche, and theories about stress relationships have been validated as factors important in a consideration of health and fitness, *awareness* alerts us to three basic ingredients in spiritual power that continue to reassert themselves. These three are and apparently always have been: *Faith, Hope,* and *Love.*

In various guises these three have been wonder cures since time began. They work wonders today. They appear to operate together as perceived by the senses. When they are experienced, they seem to operate separately but effectively, that is, a person may have *Hope* even though it may not appear that he has *Faith.* They are the charismatic components of spiritual power that, in my research among the living religions of the world, I have found convincingly demonstrated and universally employed. In their purest form, throughout the entire ecumenical system, *Faith, Hope,* and *Love* are the virtue words through which the power flows. How far their reach, how great their influence, how limitless their potential, God only knows.

We best understand the function and impact of these three components when we employ them in our own life experiences. This may be the only way that they can be empirically examined and understood. All else is objective analysis, quite inadequate for our purpose. Also, there is a good chance that if we attempt to analyze certain demonstrations of spiritual power with the instruments and conditions necessary for scientific study, we may destroy the secret signals and distort the process, impairing the desired result. It may be like asking a photographer to develop his film in the light in order to help us understand how it is done, or to insist that metamorphosis takes place outside the cocoon before we will believe the wonder-work of transmutation.

It is equally difficult to draw semantic lines between the three charismatic designations: *Faith, Hope,* and *Love.* Which comes first? Which is most important? We have been assured that "the greatest of these is *Love*," but Love has an intimate affinity with Faith and Hope.

We have also been asked to believe that "*Faith* moves mountains," and we are told that we should, "*Hope* in God, who is the health of our countenance." Yet it may be the subtle connection of all three of these components that taps the source of spiritual power, or at least provides a positive channel for its utilization.

Is it easier or better or does it really matter whether we say, "Thy sins are forgiven thee" or "Arise, take up thy bed and walk?" The point is that there is that *something* within true faith, true hope, and true love that heals. In order to discover the source and its method of expression, the impact and the flow of this subtle stream of spiritual power, one requirement is inescapable: *We must involve ourselves in the adventure.* We must come out of our physical-material world into which we have been locked by our five or more sensory perceptions and experience a rise in consciousness. In other words, we must be able not only to communicate *about* the process but to *experience* it.

Thomas E. Gaddis (1962), citing the work of Dr. Hans Selye, has noted that "the implications of his stress theory of disease . . . provide demonstration of the truth that man requires beliefs and a spiritual rootedness in order to feel happy, beautiful and well; that a knowledge *of*, not about, some areas is important; and that factors of health are rooted not in 'communication' but in *communion*."

A similar view is held by Dr. Carl Alfred Meier (1975) when he speaks of Dr. Jung's work in the field of psychology and religion: "Jung firmly believed that psychology extended beyond the realm of science into the realm of religion. He came in time to the irrevocable conclusion that the individual unconscious was rooted in a larger 'collective unconscious' which has timeless and mysterious origins and resembles many of the concepts found in Eastern religions."

Unless *we* enter into a personal exploration of spiritual

power, we are merely perpetuating what the collective unconscious has stereotyped, and a breakthrough in consciousness
is thereby thwarted. Impersonal study is nothing more than a
rendezvous with an abstract reflection. At the source of the
stream stands the inevitable challenge that an inner involvement
is necessary for an understanding of external phenomena.

To repeat, among the timeless and mysterious origins are
invariably *Faith, Hope,* and *Love* in some form, in some great
devotion, *and, always, in some involved or shared personal
relationship.*

For each of us to utilize this charismatic triad, to be aware of
it to a point where it functions reciprocally in practitioner and
patient alike, to realize that this is the bottom line of all great
achievements not only in healing but in science, religion, and
kindred disciplines may, as I have said, be the open door to our
deeper understanding of the wellspring of spiritual power. It is
not only holistic *healing* in which we are involved but holistic
living. This is the crux of the matter. We cannot give people
something we do not have, but being aware that we do have it,
as well as the will to experience and use it, gives us the courage
to chart the entire stream more thoroughly.

This assignment, then, requires a new focus and a great
tolerance for far horizons, particularly horizons of the spirit.
I recall, during the early days of my research, sharing my
thoughts about the healing demonstrations of Oral Roberts
with a physician friend. I confided to him both my doubts and
my convictions. He listened politely, nodded understandingly,
and, in deep thought, said, "No matter what we think or where
the truth lies, I would give a great deal if I could instill in my
patients the faith that these healers generate in those who come
to them."

On my return from a stay among the psychic healers of the
Philippines, I talked about the faith factor among these contro-
versial "bare-handed surgeons" to a group of doctors at the
Blackhawk Medical Society in the Midwest. I explained how
experiments had shown that when certain of these healers held
test tubes containing enzymes, the action of the enzymes was

notably accelerated. Also, there was increased electomagnetic energy when proper "communion" with their spiritual self was established. One of the members of the Society said to me, "If I had heard you talk this way about the power of belief years ago, I would have walked out on you, but lately I have begun to wonder."

He then shared an experience with me. During a busy day of surgery, he was stopped by a friend in the hospital corridor, who said to him, "Hey, Doc, when are you going to remove these warts from my hand?" The doctor replied, "Don't bother me with such trivialties. I can spoof those off." He passed his hand over the man's hand and said, "Spoof, they're gone!" A week later, the man returned and showed him his hand. The warts were gone. The man extended his other hand and said, "Spoof this one off, too!"

The attitude of the trained professional mind is not always so generous or so prepared to give healing the "light touch." It is difficult to approach, without bias or preconception, the far-out claims and the many variables to which attention needs to be given in the so-called "faith-healing" field. Certainly caution and in-depth research must be exercised, and the line between fact and fiction is often a razor's edge. Nonetheless, there should be those who are prepared to walk the edge and explore the far horizons, however distorted some may seem to be. One of holism's aims is to verify scientifically religious concepts of healing that apparently respond to laws in the still hidden psychoenergetic realm where belief plays a giant role and where *Faith, Hope,* and *Love* are more than mere placebos of the mind.

Some thirty years ago, the head of the Department of Physics, who was on my doctoral committee at the University of Iowa and who knew of my interest in parapsychology, admonished me that it was unscholarly to investigate an "isolated phenomenon." The head of Psychology at the same school was of the same opinion. When I told him of my plans to research the healing practices of the Hutterites and their "bone-setters" and the Old Order Amish and their "powwowers," it was too far out for him. Yet a local physician ventured to contribute to my study in these fields.

He had had a patient, an Amish girl, afflicted with psoriasis. She had come to him reluctantly, brought by her father in the customary horse-drawn buggy. After extended treatment, the doctor gave up and dismissed her. Several months later, a Chicago dermatologist came to the university medical center and requested "stubborn psoriasis patients" for examination and treatment. The physician drove out to see the Amish girl and discovered that she no longer had the disease. She shyly related that she had been "pow-wowed over." An Old Order Amishman, a healer, had asked her to kneel down in the backyard of her home, and they engaged in healing prayers. He then stuck a small twig from an apple tree into the ground and began "pow-wowing" with solemn German incantations and passes of his hands over his patient. Eventually, as "the spirit moved him," he intoned his emphatic "Amen" and told the girl, "In seven days the branch will be withered, and in seven days you will be healed." And in a week she *was* healed of "whatever you said I had, doctor. I never could pronounce it."

It used to be easier than it is now to become so locked into one's own specialty that one's knowledge of one particular current in the stream of healing was construed as the totality of knowledge. It is now difficult and unwise to stand by such an assumption. Holistic healing is a laboratory in which we seek, as far as possible, that which is whole, total, complete, and, also holy.

Holistic *living,* then, is the personalized process that reveals and enhances the power of holistic *healing.* As our own practice of the presence of *Faith, Hope,* and *Love* gives us a greater intimacy with the Unknown, we better understand the quest of others seeking health and wholeness, and we learn why and how they often turn to the need for spiritual power.

I continually meet people and receive letters from those who hesitate to discuss their spiritual convictions or their mystical experiences with their pastors or priests because of fear of being put down. A woman whose husband died suddenly and who was left bereft shared with me the comfort and assurance that came to her during a time of meditation when she had a vision that the spirit of her husband appeared and assured her all was well. In relating this to her minister, he first chided her for her irrationality and then advised her to see a psychiatrist. There may be questions of credibility, but there is also the need for *Faith, Hope,* and *Love* in these kinds of experiences.

There are also those who are reluctant to go to their health practitioners when they have had supernormal encounters in the healing power of *Faith, Hope,* and *Love* because they feel that the profession generally does not have an interest in or a sufficient knowledge of "mystical things." Holism recognizes that if practitioner and patient lose touch with each other, if confidence is impaired, an essential factor in healing is destroyed. Spiritual power is increased as rapport is established and as consciousness rises. There is great subtlety here, and every metaphysician is aware of it. Metaphysics suggests that patients surround the healer with light—that is, with *Faith, Hope,* and *Love*—and under such circumstances it is continually reported that, in surgical as well as nonsurgical cases, recovery is faster and that the experience of being healed has a lasting and salutary effect on the lives of both the patient *and* the practitioner.

This empathy or empathic flow rises out of a deepened sensitivity of the inner life, a proper use of meditation, and a firmer trust in the indomitable will to believe—qualities which a holistic philosophy that unites self with others and all with God is challenged to foster in the healer-and-to-be-healed equation. And all of this occurs not in any formal religious or didactic sense but by way of an innate spiritual reality that is the essence of all life.

Speculations and research about the elusive anagogic and psychic phenomena, or as some metaphysicians describe it, "spirit entities" and the interplay of the subtle body, the gross body, and the many levels of "being" from physical to etheric are all under current study and are part of the search for the meaning of life. Step by step, from ancient holistic healing on the level of its early understanding to modern psychoanalysis, psychosomatic medicine, psychosynthesis, and associated therapies, valued insight points to the need for a deeper awareness of harmonious physical, mental, and spiritual functioning.

Dramatic instances of the interplay between body-mind-spirit are continually being reported and speculated upon. Dr. A.T.W. Simeons (1962) points out:

> Cholera is caused by swallowing a microbe called a vibrio, and it is known that the cholera vibrio is highly sensitive to acids. The acid that is always present in the normal human stomach is sufficiently strong to kill the cholera vibrio almost instantly. How then does the vibrio overcome this acid barrier which separates it from the small intestines where, in the alkaline contents, it can thrive and start its murderous activity?
>
> The answer seems to be that it cannot. Only if the normal flow of acid in the stomach is shut off is the vibrio able to reach its destination. Now the one thing that stops the flow of acid in the stomach is fear and panic. So it may come about that those most terrified of death are just the ones the cholera kills, while those too young to understand the danger and those so old that life seems hardly worth living and who, fatalistically, tend to help the sick and dying around them, may survive because the secretion of their gastric juice is not emotionally inhibited. Fear might thus play an important role in the selection of victims, and in that sense it would not be incorrect to say that even in cholera psychosomatic mechanisms can be of importance."

Quite right. But the question remains: How and by what method or remedy does one conquer fear, overcome panic, or rid oneself of the terror of death over and beyond some of the attitudes cited by Dr. Simeons? This is where spiritual power properly understood, experienced, and expressed can assume its rightful role and create a new attitude of mind. This is where unique insight is required. Fears can and should be analyzed and eliminated. There are feelings of guilt the causes of which should be explored and erased. There are thoughts of death and dying that are pathological and need to be corrected. It is here that religion and science can help to discover the necessary "remedies." They will, at the same time, present a more perfect image of God as a God of love, as a channel for creative action, and as One whose children help achieve a healthier, happier, and more hopeful total life perspective. The center of participation and discovery of this kind is in the reality of *being* and the possibility of ever greater *becoming.*

Holism's efforts in these areas will inevitably create greater unity in other research projects involving the power of spiritual healing and will supply verification of such basic phenomena as prayer therapy, the laying on of hands, the value of the old admonition to "fast and pray," the practical use of mantras and affirmations, the value of meditation and silence, the influence of the "divine presence," the healing power of shrines, the efficacy of imaging health, and other fundamental but perhaps more peripheral variations and assumptions, from the most ancient to the most modern, in the metaphysical field. No matter what their differences, all believe with one accord that religion has "healing in its wings!"

One of our popular ecumenical parchments (see Figure 9–1) deals with the unanimity of belief that He Who created life continues to exercise the power to sustain that life and keep His children well!

As the holistic wings of healing unfold, the question as to where the influence of Jesus enters the scene is often asked. No religious figure has had the compelling impact of the Galilean. Christian and non-Christian alike pay respect to his titles of "Great Physician," "Master Teacher," and "Messiah."

His influence extends from the personal and intimately uttered prayer invoked "In Jesus' Name!" to the profound and poetic thoughts of Teilhard de Chardin, who insists that "Christ now invests himself organically with the very majesty of his creation."

Paleontologist Teilhard (1959), Jesuit trained and world respected, proclaims that "in a pluralistic and static Nature, the universal domination of Christ could, strictly speaking, still be regarded as an extrinsic and superimposed power. In a

Health & Healing
in the World's Great Religions

✠ CHRISTIANITY :
"The prayer of faith shall heal the sick, and the Lord shall raise him up."

CONFUCIANISM :
"High mysterious Heaven hath fullest power to heal and bind."

BUDDHISM :
"To keep the body in good health is a duty . . . otherwise we shall not be able to keep our mind strong and clear."

HINDUISM :
"Enricher, Healer of disease, be a good friend to us!"

ISLAM :
"The Lord of the worlds created me . . . and when I am sick, He healeth me."

TAOISM :
"Pursue a middle course. Thus will you keep a healthy body and a healthy mind."

SIKHISM :
"God is Creator of all, the remover of sickness, the giver of health."

JUDAISM :
"O Lord, my God, I cried to Thee for help and Thou hast healed me."

JAINISM :
"All living beings owe their present state of health to their own Karma."

ZOROASTRIANISM:
"Love endows the sick body of man with firmness and health."

BAHA'I :
"All healing comes from God."

SHINTO :
"Foster a spirit that regards both good and evil as blessings, and the body spontaneously becomes healthy."

THE FELLOWSHIP FOR SPIRITUAL UNDERSTANDING, P.O. Box 816, Palos Verdes Estates, California 90274
© 1972   Phone: (213) 373-2669

spiritually converging world this *Christic* energy acquires an urgency and intensity of another order altogether . . . and it is in no way metaphorical to say that man finds himself capable of now experiencing and discovering his God in the whole length, breadth and depth of the world in movement."

My feeling about the role of Jesus Christ in the discovery and utilization of spiritual power in holistic healing is that there is both a minimum and an extended view. Credit for the term "minimum view" must go to John Noss, who introduced the term in a footnote to his monumental work, *Man's Religions* (1972):

> The healing miracles of Jesus as preserved for us in tradition may present many difficulties, but if we could speak of a minimum view, it would be something like this: in a world like that of Jesus' time, where spiritual and nervous tensions were so great, there must have been many instances of functional disorders, greatly aggravated by fears and repressions and exhibiting many of the symptoms of organic diseases among all classes of the people. The nobility of Jesus' own faith mediated through a wholesome, sympathetic and challenging personality, remade their faith and caused their alarming symptoms to vanish instantly. To this minimum view a great deal might be added.

Fair enough! And a great deal *is* added by those who insist that this humanistic view is subminimal, that Jesus was considerably more than a moral and ethical exemplar or master sympathizer or mesmerist or wonder-worker or psychoanalyst. They are persuaded that He was a foreordained manifestation of God Who demonstrated the miracles and mysteries that those who truly follow Him may also perform. They also believe that He did even "greater things," because He returned to the Father, leaving the Holy Spirit active and influential in the world at large.

Whether one takes a minimum or maximum view, the fact remains that Jesus' holistic approach to life inspired a phenomenal confidence in the power of spiritual healing. Through Him, just as through the great prophets and avatars of other faiths, the hidden potential of the *integrated triad* (Bach, 1977), body-mind-spirit, became a channel for the *charismatic triad, Faith, Hope,* and *Love* and helped us to recognize, as has been said, that it is not only holistic healing but holistic *living* to which we must give personal and undivided attention.

Holistic *healing,* as we have seen, is the movement in society bringing together working teams in the health care field and outlining new, united paths to well-being, fitness, and fullness of life.

Holistic *living* is the movement within the individual, in healer and patient alike, a self-dedicated adventure to which each person must be committed sincerely.

Cooperatively, holistic healing and holistic living create the new and needed awareness that *responsibility for your health lies within yourself and that Faith, Hope,* and *Love* are factors in the process. The holistic movement is designed to help us, and our responsibility to help ourselves will inextricably help *it.* It represents a unique new camaraderie between the healing arts and the individual, and one of its strongest and most significant links is its interspiritual understanding of the total person.

The full force of this united emphasis is still in the making, but, as has been said, a rare adventure in the ecumenicity of "Spirit" is under way. The combined search for the source and the flow of healing is one in which religions of the world can conscientiously cooperate and by means of which the skills, knowledge, and experiences of the exact sciences and the humanities, of church leaders and laity, of traditionalists and people of the "new age," can make their contributions to the power of total living in the life of our time.

There is considerable evidence that nourishment of the spirit is related to body health and performance. We have seen how the common denominators of Faith, Hope, and Love are expressions of the spiritual power available to us. Certain spiritual activities may cause anatomical as well as functional modifications of tissues and organs. These phenomena are sometimes observed through a state of prayer, not as a mechanical recitation of words but rather as an elevation of consciousness that both permeates and transcends our world. It is not an intellectual state but one which is experiential in nature. The power of this consciousness in the healing process has been reported throughout history. The cases recorded by the Medical Bureau at Lourdes testify to the influence of prayer on pathological conditions.

Julian Byrd conveys his warm, sensitive understanding as he describes his experiences of the support derived from spiritual sharing that heals all who experience such feelings together.

10

Spiritual Help in Health Care

JULIAN BYRD, S.T.M.

There is a Power and a Presence that pervades this Universe and all within it. This Presence is life and Its power is love, within and through which we identify and upon which we call at various times to assist us through crises or to guide us to new heights. I choose to call this Presence and Power *God*.

During my years of ministry as chaplain, first at M.D. Anderson Hospital, the Cancer Research Institution for the University of Texas System in Houston, and now at Hermann Hospital, also a major hospital within the Texas Medical Center, I have become more aware of the pervading presence of spirit within each of us. This essence is not always recognized consciously or intentionally called upon for aid. Rather, I believe it exists as a natural resource to be used for support when things get rough and for leadership when things are going well. In my work with patients, this may be as simple a thing as looking at the dynamics of a patient's family and identifying the members who most portray those qualities needed at certain times. Each of us, when challenged, may automatically call upon that which we know best or feel strongly will bring us forth into more peace of mind and renewal, both of body and soul. When reserves appear to be exhausted, when body is weary, heart heavy, and hope diminished, more often than not we find a way to accept, to go forward, and to become replenished. There are as many techniques and theological methods and beliefs for this type of uplifting as there are individual personalities. I have found that my awareness of this spirit of being within me and working through me has been the determining factor in helping others to find the resources of their faith that will aid them, both uniquely and personally.

This entire subject of spiritual resources and meeting crises is not easily documented. One of the ways to understand the process is to observe how persons, in periods of tragedy and disillusionment, fall back on whatever strengths they happen to have or can mobilize at the time. Only, in most people with whom I have worked, it appears that this reaction is not a conscious one or a strictly thought-through response but is more intuitive, more spontaneous. Some, however, often do not know that their answer is within their faith, within themselves. Perhaps even with this realization, there is hesitancy to get in touch with and respond with that awareness. The presence of a minister may promote freedom, not necessarily through his words but perhaps simply because the patient perceives a oneness of spirit between them that brings comfort, strength, creativity.

The need is great to identify who we are and what it is we are expressing and why. Tracing this kind of thinking in my own life, I recall when I first began working at M.D. Anderson Hospital in 1958. I was a young man with a year's parish experience as a pastor and a couple of years' training in an institutional setting as a chaplain. I discovered very soon that I was limited in being able to tap my emotional and spiritual reserves. After visiting with the young cancer patients in the pediatric unit of the hospital, I would leave feeling very depressed and discouraged; I would sometimes avoid going back. A number of times I caught myself feeling guilty because I had not gone back to see a family or a patient in that unit for a while, just because I dreaded it. I wasn't able to clearly identify why.

Having come up through the academic system, where you don't reveal your flaws unless you have to, I was unaccustomed to admitting my weaknesses. I was trained to present a strong, adequate front—perhaps all of us have been taught to do this from our earlier years. A part of it was who I was as an individual even before I got into school, so I can't blame it all on the academic system. I had a need to please and to be accepted that made it difficult for me to say, "I don't feel like I have what it takes."

I soon began to recognize, though, that it did help to talk with other people about what I was feeling and experiencing. Sharing with others became a resource available to me that I often called upon. In using this technique, I discovered that one of the things I was doing with the young cancer patients was overidentifying with their parents. Our children were very young at the time, and, frequently, the children I was seeing were the same ages as my son and daughter. It was very easy for me to become attached to the parents and to take upon myself the strain they were feeling. I had to get to a point where I could handle this.

Once I learned that I could talk to somebody and get a greater understanding of myself and, consequently, gain an increased ability to meet the challenges of my profession, I could consciously make the decision to do it whenever I began to feel inadequate. I found that I was not alone in my doubts about being able to say something helpful to the patients and to their families. Nurses experienced similar fears and reactions. Physicians also reached points in their lives when they could not go and talk with their patients. Initially, I was reluctant to discuss my inner emotions, because this was so new for me. But, as I began to be more open with myself and with others, I learned in my prayers with God to admit, "I don't have it any more, God. What's the matter? Why is it that every time I run into this kind of situation I feel so inadequate? Come on,

God, give me a hand." This *was* new—to be able to communicate to God the true expression of my feelings. It was through the recognition that I needed help that I developed an honest relationship with God and began to accept myself.

A couple of social workers on the hospital staff assisted me greatly in finding my own self-direction. They were considerably older than I was; both had a lot of maturity and a lot of experience. They helped me, first of all, to identify what was going on within myself, and, then, they led me to give expression to those thoughts and feelings. They even acknowledged that, with all their maturity, experience, and training, they, too, had times when they felt defeated, when their resources appeared exhausted, and when they had to reach out. They also shared their seeking experiences with me. This brought me into a greater understanding of our oneness, for we each have the power to choose change and to remove the blocks to our awareness of the Presence of God active within our lives.

In my life's work, this realization brought forth more effective techniques in working with patients. There were things I could do to adjust. For instance, I began scheduling my time so that I spent anywhere from an hour to an hour and a half in the pediatric unit. Then, I would deliberately leave and go to visit patients somewhere else. Even though all the people I was seeing were cancer patients, I found that I was better able to interact with the adult patients than with the children and their parents. Certainly, there were many times in working with the adult patients that I became discouraged and depressed, too; but I could feel differently about myself and my abilities in assisting them than I did with the younger patients. Upon returning to the pediatric unit, I did not feel so defeated, so completely exhausted. My energies were revitalized, and my inner boundaries were not so confining.

I became attuned to the reality that what is within me, the spirit and essence of me, will sustain me. As a result of acknowledging my deep needs and calling forth the powers of God within, what was most meaningful for me came through my thinking and feeling. I have found this to be true in dealing with patients and their families. In many thousands of counseling sessions, I have observed one common denominator: a search for meaning. We need answers and a better way. Many come to realize that the answers do come from within, from knowing themselves and from getting in touch with who they are. Each of us has to have his or her own experience with a spiritual self in order to come to this realization. Although the needs of patients and their families may be obvious to *me,* their answers come through *their* seekings. I make myself available to them so that their questions may flow more freely, but their adjustment comes from within the resources of their faith rather than because of anything I personally say or do.

During those early years, the view I had held of my ministry changed drastically. Previously, I had considered the ministry as a channel for giving, or for bringing, to others something that they did not already have. I began to discover that the Holy Spirit was way ahead of me, though. I didn't necessarily introduce people to God or to their faith; but somehow, in our interactions, there were times when they became more aware of the wellsprings of their faith, of their indwelling spirit, even in the midst of crises. This is a dynamic process, with no obviously converging points of recognition in time or place. It is a happening which brings alarming awareness, at times, and it is always a basis from which to grow into a new consciousness.

Perhaps it is most accurate to state that a person's faith is an instrument for health. Healing, as commonly interpreted, implies the restoration of right relationships—the cure of moral, physical, intellectual, and emotional disturbances. We are concerned with the one entity, the human being. In reality, there is no separation of mind, body, and spirit. We generally think of specialists in medicine, such as psychiatrists and psychologists, as addressing problems of the mind; of physicians in a number of areas taking care of the physical needs of the body; and of pastors, priests, and rabbis ministering to the needs of the spirit. Each of us, lay person and professional alike, needs to recognize that when working with an individual whose wholeness is broken, our task as healers is to facilitate the movement toward health in totality.

As a minister in the traditional Christian framework, I have witnessed states of health being replaced by illness, and I have observed natural stages of development in the uniqueness of a person being somewhat delayed or arrested. I have found myself facilitating the process of harmony within individuals by being present with them and allowing their inner feelings and inner thoughts to flow uninterrupted, so that what they are in the process of becoming is free to be and to go forward. The need is to address people in whatever circumstance they find themselves and to assist them in moving from brokenness to wholeness, from illness to health, from arrested growth and development to a fuller, more creative expression of who they really are. It is important for the one being treated or counseled to know that what he is expressing, feeling, and being is a step in conscious evolution toward becoming a whole person.

Oftentimes, patients may feel as though God, as they understand Him, has let them down. They may have been very active church members during their adult years, and they may have attempted to live the kind of lives that they felt were in keeping with Christian principles. Consequently, they may have begun to wonder what they have done to deserve the pain and suffering of their present conditions. Faith, in this type of situation, has become equated with a kind of protection or insurance against anything tragic happening to them. Because they are ill, they are disappointed or disillusioned because the faith they presumed would protect them has failed.

"Faithful" persons who find themselves as patients may also begin to have doubts and uncertainties about their own prognoses or even about how closely God may be involved with them at this time of suffering. They may have the idea that to discuss, or to even think about, doubts and uncertainties, much less give expression to lack of faith, will be viewed harshly by God. Indeed, they may think they will be punished further. The recognition that the expression of feelings, including doubts, may be a way of mobilizing faith resources has escaped consciousness. Somehow, they have to be helped to see that faith and doubt play hide-and-seek in the believer's heart throughout life. I have yet to meet a person of faith who has not at some moments been haunted by uncertainties or a person proclaiming atheism or expressing skepticism who has not at times acknowledged seeds of faith.

We are all challenged to realize and to actualize more fully the potentials of our uniqueness in more positive ways and to accept responsibility for the management of our own lives. In dealing with those who are physically incapacitated, I have found the inner working of the self overshadows the apparent infirmity. So many thoughts come to a patient in addition to the hope of physical repair.

In the late 1950s and early 1960s, before the issue of integration had reached its full impact upon the South and when we were still practicing the rigid traditions of racial separateness, we conducted interfaith worship services in the Pathology Department conference room at M.D. Anderson. There were many Sunday mornings when I walked up the ramp to the front of the hospital feeling, "What am I doing here? What have I got to say to these people?" I never went there without a prepared manuscript, yet frequently I wondered whether what I had to say would really be helpful. I wondered how I could assist them when, after all, they taught me so much as I worked with them. I can honestly say, though, that I never left the hospital after the services were over on Sunday when I did not feel elated. At times, it was almost as though I were walking right off the platform in front of the hospital, my feet not even touching the ground.

Except for this coming together each Sunday morning, all facilities throughout the hospital were segrated—black and white, male and female. On every floor, in every location, there were separate restrooms, side-by-side drinking fountains; there were separate cafeterias, and an isolated wing of the hospital for black patients. The physicians, however, did serve together. But the only really integrated experience was to be found in these worship services. Here was a feeling of oneness, at-one-ment.

One Sunday morning, a rather elderly white lady was wheeled into the service. I had met her before the service began and had talked with her briefly, along with some of the other patients who were there. Before the formal order of the service, I was leading the congregation in singing. A black lady was wheeled in by one of the volunteers and was parked beside the white lady. The white lady held out her hymnal, and the two of them shared the hymnal and sang together. The service continued with reading of Scripture. Then I noticed that the white lady was beginning to cry. During the meditation, she began crying even more. One of the volunteers, noticing and being sensitive to her needs, wheeled her out. After the services, I went to see her to offer my assistance and to find out what had made her cry. When I entered the room, I found her discussing the episode with her roommate, and she seemed a bit surprised to see me. I told her that I had observed her crying during the worship service and had wanted to come by to see how she was.

What she said, in effect, was that she had been an active church member all her life and had frequently attended services. But this was the first time she had ever been in a service where a black person was present. She said, "This morning I was sitting there. We were singing, and this person was wheeled in and parked by me. I rather spontaneously, without even thinking, extended my hymnal for her to sing with me. Then I realized she was black. I was caught, then. I was just kind of in shock, but I didn't dare withdraw my hymnal. This black person began singing with me! I began to get really emotionally shaken, because I recognized my own prejudice. I never thought that I would worship anywhere with a black person; and here I was, not only worshiping with one, but sharing my hymnal with one. I was just so unnerved by it; and I felt, 'Why, she's a Child of God, too, and we are worshiping the same God.' And I couldn't overcome all those feelings I've had for all of these years. So, I just got more and more unnerved by it and started crying more and the volunteer wheeled me out."

"Now," she said, "I have to face the fact that blacks are God's children the same as I am, and that doesn't help me to get rid of my prejudice right away. But it does help me to recognize that we are brothers and sisters. I'll never be able to go to church again and feel quite the same way I did before this."

The experience of worshiping together in that setting was one that caused a lot of people to stretch their boundaries. They may not all have had racial prejudices, but almost everyone came from a different denomination or faith background. It was not uncommon at all to have patients express new awareness after coming to these worship services. Their feeling was, "We have this in common—all of us are cancer patients and we are all Children of God. Whatever differences we have in theology are minor compared to what we have in common." This type of community experience within the health care facility is not private or pietistic but filled with faith and knowing that the resources of that community are there to help the total well-being of the individual.

Being with a person is central and first. What we do while we are there is secondary. Techniques and skills are important, of course, and necessary in facilitating awareness of the inner spirit at times. But the essential thing is being available in the relationship with someone else. When you are really with a person, that "being there" is more effective than methods used when you are not in tune with the "who" of the person seeking aid. If we are really caring and are concerned for someone, that makes the difference, that helps them. Jesus said "For where two or three are gathered together in my name, there am I in the midst of them." (Matthew 18:20). When there is genuine care or valuing, there is recognition of an ultimate dimension to the relationship. For me, God is present. The Holy Spirit is present.

Most of us place our greatest emphasis on what we are going to do next, what we are going to do when we get off work this afternoon, and what we are going to do tonight. We wonder what we are going to do when we get the house or the car paid for, what we are going to do when we graduate, or what we are going to do when the children grow up and leave home. Secondarily, we think, "Who am I? What is the meaning of my life? What am I about?" These kinds of identity questions, the "Who am I?" questions, are not given so much prominence as the action questions. Yet, in traditional Christianity, the Master Teacher Jesus always placed emphasis on the "who" rather than on the "what." Perhaps in relating to a patient, a friend, a loved one, and, most importantly, to ourselves, we need to seek the answer to the "who." We may then find that who we are in a healing situation, our own or someone else's, is permanent and lasting and that the "what" of our experience is secondary.

We must all search for answers that fit our unique needs. We are such creative, intelligent beings that we can find just the right answer to fit our perplexities; whether or not they are in common with the doctrines and ways of others does not matter. In seeking, each finds his or her own self-direction.

As an extension of its emergency facilities, Hermann Hospital incorporated the Life-Flight Helicopter service in 1976. Three helicopters, carrying a doctor and a nurse aboard each, operate twenty-four hours a day within a 130-mile radius of Houston to transport injured persons quickly to the hospital. The Life-Flight Helicopter will respond immediately to any authorized call in case of an accident, whether the severity of injuries is known or not. Such was the case within the last year when our helicopter brought in a young man who had been involved in an automobile accident.

I was called early that morning to come to the emergency unit, as the injured boy had died en route to the hospital. I was to meet the family, who would be following, and to be with them as they learned of his death.

The youth who was fatally injured had been driving the car when it went out of control. His older stepbrother and step-father were passengers in the same vehicle, but they had escaped without injury and were brought to Hermann Hospital by a passerby at the scene of the accident. Upon their arrival, they learned of the boy's death and were, needless to say, very shaken and distraught. The stepbrother was in shock. He could not express anything.

The stepfather called his wife. He told her that there had been an accident and that her son was at the hospital. He waited until she arrived at the hospital before telling her of the boy's death. Since it took her almost two hours to get to the emergency unit, she had many moments to consider the seriousness of the situation, and she was ashen as she walked through the hospital doors. I met her and escorted her through the corridors to the private room where her husband was waiting. They met and embraced. She sensed what she was going to hear, but, of course, she did not want to know what had really happened. He told her that her son was dead. She immediately went through denial, "No, it can't be!" Her emotions were rampant and her acceptance nonexistent. We spent some time with her there in that room during this difficult period. I was trying to just be present with her, to facilitate what was going on, to be reassuring in any way I could. But, of course, initially, there was no way to be reassuring.

As she began to fully express her trauma, she identified me as a minister. She recognized that I was there with her and that she could talk with me, just as she had talked with the others in the room. She said that she couldn't accept her son's death, that it just couldn't be true, that God had told her only recently in a direct communique that her son was going to be a minister. Some days later, she related, the son had told her that he had had the same revelation from God, quite independent of her experience. She could not fathom why, if God wanted him to be a minister, He would take him now. She began to incorporate some of her own theology into the situation, and I simply allowed her the freedom to reach within herself for whatever she needed at the moment. It was essential, at this point, that she use the resources of her own faith; it was not important what the reasoning was or whether anyone else in the room understood her or agreed with her. She drew upon the strength she had for her own special answers, for her own self-direction, and, from her own resources, comfort and a different kind of hope began for her.

We went to the chapel and spent another hour there praying together. I continued to be with her, to assist her in verbalizing her feelings, to help her see that she could question God about all of this. She chose to affirm that God would help her to handle this. I knew, too, that her life and the lives of the other family members would also be enriched as a result of this experience, not by the tragic loss, but by the entire life happening and the sharing within the midst of this crisis.

Some months passed, and I received a lengthy, handwritten letter from this lady. She expressed her belief that God had used her son's death to lead a lot of other people to Him. Many of the classmates of the stepbrother who had survived were traumatized by this whole event and began to visit in her home often. A community of caring developed. According to her, a number of these young people found a connection with their spiritual selves as a result of her son's death and of their experience throughout the crisis. She needed this type of specific, concrete evidence that her son's death had brought about good. This is calling on the resources of your faith. It is turning to what you believe and affirming what you are experiencing as real.

The manner in which faith is called upon in crises is different for each person. The important thing is its effectiveness. Another patient, a young woman, had been involved in an automobile accident with her husband and two infant children. She was unconscious for a period of time as a result of the accident. Her husband had been killed instantly, as were her two children. I was called to be with the family, and I ministered to the parents of the deceased husband and to the patient's mother. Together, we had the task of telling this young woman, after she regained consciousness, that she was left without a family. That was hard—hard for all of us.

Then, we began twice daily sessions of grief counseling over the next few weeks and before she was discharged. She had been an active person in the church in her youth, and she was able, in this situation, to call upon her faith in God and her belief in life after death, and to find strength and meaning there that helped her put the pieces back together. She was able to give expression to all of her doubts, all of her uncertainties. She was angry that this had happened, and she addressed that anger to the driver of the other vehicle, who had run a stop sign. She was angry at the disruption of her life and toward God for having permitted this to happen. She never accused God of causing it to happen, but she did feel that He could have stepped in and kept it from happening. My task was to help her to give expression to all she was experiencing—to all the fears—and to get in touch with and identify a basis for going forward from this point.

Before she left the hospital, she began to know that she was going to have to do some radical reorienting of her life. She did not want to return to her home, for even though she had begun to reconcile herself to her husband's death, it was much more difficult to adapt to the children's deaths. She dreamed about them; they were alive for her. She was afraid that she would be unable to walk into the home she had shared with them, see their toys and clothes, and remain at least somewhat composed. One day, when she realized a friend of hers was coming to visit with her in the hospital and was bringing her young daughter, the patient panicked. She did not want the child to visit. We talked about this, and she finally agreed to let the little girl come. This young, now childless mother held her friend's daughter in her arms and cried.

I continued to see her as an outpatient. She soon left her wheelchair and became ambulatory again. She sold her home and moved back to a different part of town. She had been a school teacher until after she was married, and she was able to resume that profession. With a lot of support from her family and friends, and by calling upon her faith, she continued life. Through her prayers, she affirmed her faith in God and asked for His help. Her movement through this entire ordeal was never like putting a patch on things, though. So often, well-meaning persons say, "You've got to get hold of yourself; you're a person of faith; your faith will sustain you; you've got to be strong; if you believe in God, then trust Him to help you through this." It's all right to say, "Trust God," but it is quite another thing to put the lid on feelings, to try to help an individual by stifling the expression of who he or she is and what he or she is experiencing as real.

It is through the expression of all we are that we get in touch with the qualities of spirit that are within and available to us at all times.

Often, if no expression is given to feelings or to all that is going on within, the flow of spirit is blocked. The helping person (the physician, the nurse, the pastor, the friend, the family member) who is interacting facilitates the sorting and putting together of pieces by allowing the other person to shout, to come unglued—if that is what it takes. The essence of spirit is there working within the individual; cooperating with this activity brings harmony. The feeling that somebody cares, is willing to get involved, and is not himself afraid of intense feelings aids the patient in arriving at new answers, better ways, and more meaningful insights. To trust this spirit within promotes the rebirth of wholeness.

While chaplain at Anderson, I got to know quite well a couple from another state who were in their early sixties. The man came to the hospital as a cancer patient and handled his terminal illness very well. He and his wife, both persons of faith, helped each other greatly during this difficult time. Two years after his death, the wife returned as a cancer patient. Only now she was struggling and was filled with a great many doubts. Uncertain that she would be able to handle it by herself, she questioned God's goodness and mercy and could not understand why this was happening or what it was all about. These are questions that all of us ask at one time or another, but she was verbalizing them now.

Prayer circles were formed around the world for this lady, and many reached out in love to her. Her home community rallied in support. Her daughter, a social worker, and I talked together to find ways in which she could be helpful. An Episcopal priest who practiced faith healing was called upon and visited the patient. I was asked if I would participate in a healing service at the patient's bedside. We all discussed this, and each of us reached an understanding of what we considered healing to be. For me, I believe God can and does heal, and I expressed this to everyone present. I added that healing, within my philosophy, is much broader than physical restoration. My concept of healing encompasses the return to wholeness that once was felt, regardless of what has happened to the body, the feeling of being at peace and in oneness. I told the patient that I was interested in seeing her be able to communicate with her daughter in such a way that they could share life's experiences each day in a meaningful way. She understood that my prayer for her health would be for more than the removal of physical disease alone.

We had the healing service, a first for me. The priest prayed for recovery of her physical body and the ridding of cancer. Then I prayed, including affirmations of total well-being.

Interestingly enough, this patient did have a rather spontaneous physical recovery. She was able to get out of bed and was wheeled outside to sit under the trees each day. Her spirits were buoyed, and she felt she was getting well. She really felt, and perhaps hoped, too, that the cancer was going away. The beautiful thing was that, in spite of the fact that the disease only regressed temporarily and did not go away, she did not return to all the doubts and uncertainties about her own worthwhileness, about her relationship to God. She displayed a spirit of congeniality and assistance that helped other people who came to see her. She expressed deep gratitude for all she had come to realize and recognize during those last days. Prayers were openly shared. Nothing was held back, for there was no longer anything of which to be afraid. She talked openly about what she was going through. It was a very triumphant experience. Healing had occurred. It was there for anyone to see who has witnessed the process, but it was not a physical healing. She touched upon the reality of her true nature, and there was calm that went beyond the *appearances* of lack and imperfection.

So it is that even in contemplating death we can become aware of our true being. Although we see death as the termination of the body, we can be in touch with that terminal part and still recognize that it is not the end of life, as many of us fear. Rather, when we are in tune with the whole of life, we recognize this thing called death as a process in the universal plan. We are progressing from one stage to another. From this perspective, fear begins to fade. Knowing that there is a higher level, that there is more than just this one life, we begin to achieve a greater sense of peace and confidence as we arrive at that moment of transition.

Spiritual healing is available to all, and it does occur. It may not always be named that, but it is there. It is real evidence of the working of God's Spirit within our lives. My major role as Chaplain is to help others to recognize this Presence within themselves; and, for me, it is consistent with the psychologist's or psychiatrist's understanding of the resources of personality that an individual can call upon. Such a specialist identifies psychological strengths. That is no different, in terms of concrete expression, than identifying the Spirit at work. There is just a different language to talk about the same kind of human experience.

We all must know and understand ourselves as well as possible in order to help one another—and to help ourselves. Our ability to help is in direct proportion to our being in touch with all of our own emotional and spiritual dynamics. Otherwise, we may find ourselves, a good bit of the time, attempting to meet as many of our own needs as possible rather than meeting the ones of the person who has come seeking to mend a shambled state. Of course, none of us can ever get to the point where we know ourselves completely or know exactly how to call forth the Spirit within, for we are always progressing in our growth experiences. But we learn more about it if we are attentive and recognize who we really are in what we are presently doing. There are so many ways. A primary part of the process is to know what our own limitations are and where our own strengths and assets are.

We need to know our own defense systems and how we are using them. People who work in hospitals have many such "protective" techniques. The doctor can, if he chooses, use the stethoscope at times to distance himself emotionally from a patient. If checking the heart or blood pressure, it is easy to get by without conversing, because something is being done for the patient. The clergyman can use his official garb to get him into a lot of places. At the same time, that reversed collar can be used as a device to stay detached from the patient; it can be a symbol of a very busy person who can only stay a minute. Never sitting down communicates to the patient that the person visiting really does not want to be there or does not have much time for him. The danger in these defense techniques is that they heighten the sense of isolation that the patient who may be dying is already experiencing. The rejection is deeply felt. So, if we are going to be truly helpful and feel good about our roles within the health care field, it is crucial that we participate in the process through our own self-awareness and self-understanding. Through these dynamics, we begin to know when to say "no," when to say "yes"—and still be helpful.

There are times when we all use our defense systems, but we need to *know* we are doing it and not pretend. We need to be genuine in our concern and caring for the patient, and we need to be honest when we aren't willing to get in there and mix it up with them. In acknowledging our boundaries and working within them until they are expanded, we can be of much greater assistance, both to those in need and to ourselves.

This is a life-long process—getting to know oneself. It is not to be hurried and pressed forward prematurely, nor is it wise to live in the past. Rather, as we experience life from moment to moment and stay in the conscious now, we can begin to feel the rhythm of the universe and the order of life. This harmony of being is within and throughout everything; it sustains and supports us even without our naming it. Awareness of this powerful order of things can promote wholeness. We each have an individual responsibility to seek our inner cadence and to give it full expression in our lives, which is vital to our physical, mental, and spiritual well-being.

We have traced illness to stress, and we have seen how the response to stress depends upon the perception of each individual, upon the way he sees the world. Sickness, then, eventually starts in the mind. Therefore, it is the mind that needs healing. The aim is to help a person abandon his deluded ideas that the world of dis-tress he experiences is real rather than a product of his own belief about himself. People who need help are in some way attacking themselves, and, frequently, they will regard their behavior as "self-destructive." Until they begin to question their belief system, the thoughts they think are real, and begin to separate truth from illusions, very little progress may be made to reduce the stress in their lives.

Dr. Knight is a unique combination of physician, psychiatrist, and clergyman who brings an integrated perspective to the awareness that every therapeutic relationship that works provides for a healing of both parties and inevitably includes a spiritual dimension—whether or not it is so labeled.

11

Spiritual Psychotherapy and Self-Regulation

JAMES A. KNIGHT, M.D.

In a broad sense, psychotherapy is a religious quest—a quest for meaning. Whatever form psychotherapy may take, it must allow the person to transcend his own human predicament, to find continuity, and to come to believe that he is part of a whole greater than himself. Whether the end result is called health, salvation, or peace of mind, the new condition must allow the person to come to grips with his real human-ness, to find relief from the pangs of guilt, and to experience forgiveness and love. Something of the significance of the term "health" in the Bible may be gathered from the one Hebrew cognate that translates both health (*shalem*) and peace (*shalom*).

A MINISTRY OF HEALING

A young man, Charmides, in one of Plato's dialogues, complains about a headache. He wants a particular drug, but Socrates explains to him at length that this simple treatment is not adequate. To treat the head by itself, apart from the body as a whole, he says, is utter folly. The ideal approach had been described to Socrates by a Thracian physician:

> You ought not to attempt to cure eyes without head,
> Or head without body,
> So you should not treat body
> Without soul.

The totality of human need cannot be met when people try to compartmentalize the person into body, soul, or psyche; the person's needs are best met when he is seen as a whole person and when all of the resources of humankind and God are appropriated to meet those needs.

Healing power is latent in the person because it is latent in the nature of things. We live in a universe where positive values are actualized through an interplay of natural, human, and divine creativity. Every therapist counts on the drive for recovery, deep within his patient, that goes beyond the conscious devising of himself and his patients. The therapist's task is to participate in the releasing of healing processes rather than to invent them.

Everyone involved in healing should accept the premise that healing comes from God. A French surgeon of the sixteenth century, Ambroise Paré, expressed this concept in memorable words: "God heals the wound; I merely dress it." The surgeon, in the care of the wound, cleanses it, removes the debris, and brings together the edges of the skin. Most of what he does is to remove the obstacles to healing. He is not the source of healing, and he knows more about the obstacles to healing than about healing itself. Even in psychotherapy, much of what we do relates to removing the psychological obstacles to healing, for the healing itself comes from God, regardless of by what name He is called.

In every individual, there is an attempt to be healed. In treatment, the therapist tries to strengthen the healing dimensions in the patient. Although the cleansing and dressing of a psychological wound may include some dimensions not considered by the surgeon, the recognition of God as the source of all healing will help us keep our efforts in the proper perspective, regardless of the professional disciplines we represent.

There is no hierarchy of healing. When we see in perspective our participation in the healing process, many sibling problems among healing groups will be eliminated. Each of us can then bring to bear our professional skills, our gifts of self (the individual person as an instrument of healing), and our organization, (for example, the group life of the church) in the healing of the sick person.

Healing is holy. Can anything be holier than helping one who asks for help? When two work together for healing, God is there. *Vocatus atque non vocatus Deus aberit:* "Invited, even not invited, God is present." Although many varieties of psychotherapy may accept this statement as true, the recognition and acknowledgment of His presence may permit His influence to be more easily felt and heeded. Such a recognition should, in no sense, lead the therapist to confuse himself with God.

In order to broaden our understanding of healing, we should look at the art and practice of healing as described in the New Testament. In studying the Biblical healing stories, one discovers several basic conditions operative in almost all of the cases described.

First, the healing takes place through the activity of an individual or a group who are perceived as having the authority and power to heal. In most cases, both the healer and the one being healed share this conviction as to the authority and power of the healer. In those cases in which the one being healed is skeptical or agnostic, there are significant other persons in his environment who do credit the healing person or persons with authority and power.

Second, the act of healing often includes the recital of previous healings or other divine events that manifest power for wholeness and transformation. Mircea Eliade (1949), in *The Sacred and the Profane,* emphasizes that primitive man, in his healing rites, sought healing through the regeneration of the sources of his life, with which he made contact through the ritual recitation of the story of creation. The sick man symbolically became *contemporary* with the "creation" and became well because he began life over again with his reserve of vital forces intact, as it was at the moment of his birth.

Third, in the New Testament healing stories, the healing action came in response to the initiative and request of the sick person, his friends, or his relatives. Active desire and expectancy permeated the healing situation. By the pool of Bethesda, before the healing took place, Jesus asked the man if he truly wanted to be healed (John 5:1–16).

Leslie Weatherhead (1952) maintains that a fundamental element in all the healing stories is the quality of "expectant trust." Jerome Frank, in *Persuasion and Healing* (1974), shows expectant trust to be the central thread woven through all the healing practices of man, both ancient and modern. The many occasions on which Jesus states that the faith or expectancy of the sick person has been the fundamental instrumentality of the healing do serve to underline how absolutely essential this element seems to have been for the healings of the New Testament and the early church.

Fourth, healing seems to have taken place almost invariably in some corporate context. In his ministry, Jesus was almost always surrounded by crowds of people. An example of this is the story of the sick man who had to be let down through the roof into the room where Jesus was because the door was blocked by large numbers of people (Mark 2:1–5). This story is especially significant because it appears to have been the friends and not the patient himself who sought the healing and had the expectant trust. The group atmosphere in the New Testament healing episodes was a most significant factor in the preparation and support of the healing process. In the life of the early church, where healing became more and more associated with the corporate worship and the sacramental life of the believing community, the element of group atmosphere became a factor of major importance.

Fifth, in many of the instances of Biblical healing, the healer employs suggestion and authoritative verbal direction as an important part of his method. Jesus used this approach. Often, this suggestive element was simply the communication of the firm assumption that the ill person would be healed of the illness.

Sixth, in many of the Biblical stories, physical materials and means were used as an instrumental aspect of the healing action. These included saliva for the stammering tongue, clay for the eyes, the laying on of hands, the anointing with oil, or the symbolic cleansing with water—all used to effect healing. In the early church, the Eucharist, anointing with oil, and baptism were the three major occasions of healing, according to Origen and others.

FROM DECEPTION TO REALITY

Unfortunately, some so-called psychotherapy is no more than the therapist and patient sharing one another's illusions. Unless psychotherapy moves far beyond this, there can be no healing for patient or psychotherapist.

The major task of psychotherapy is to help the patient see that much of what he views as reality is actually illusion. The blocks to truth must be removed. Nowhere is the Biblical adage more relevant: "Ye shall know the truth and the truth shall make you free." The patient begins to abandon his fixed delusional system when he comes to grips with the spurious cause and effect relationships on which it rests. He reverses his thinking and understands that the world he thought projected its effects on him were effects made by his projections on the world. Psychotherapy does not establish reality but makes way for reality.

Psychotherapy must confront illusions. As succinctly stated in *Psychotherapy: Purpose, Process and Practice* (1976):

> A madman will defend his own delusions because in them he sees his own salvation. Thus, he will attack the one who tries to save him from them, believing that he is attacking them. This curious circle of attack-defense is one of the most difficult problems with which the psychotherapist must deal. In fact, this is his central task; the core of psychotherapy. The therapist is seen as one who is attacking the patient's most cherished possession; his picture of himself. And since this picture has become the patient's security as he perceives it, the therapist cannot but be seen as a real source of danger, to be attacked and even killed.

A clear example of the way a person's picture of himself is attacked in a healing context and the consequences thereof is presented in Victor Hugo's *Les Miserables*. Jean Valjean, the exconvict newly released from a long prison sentence, underwent a dramatic change in his personality because of the overwhelming and unexpected kindness of the bishop whom he had robbed of six silver plates and had even contemplated killing.

Jean Valjean felt dimly that the pardon of this priest was the hardest assault and the most formidable attack that he had yet sustained, and that his hardness of heart would be complete if it resisted this kindness. If he yielded, he must renounce that hatred with which the acts of other men had for so many years filled his soul, and in which he found satisfaction. This time, he must conquer or be conquered. The struggle, a gigantic and decisive struggle, had begun between his own egocentric self and the goodness of the bishop.

The bishop radiated goodness and kindness. Jean Valjean's projections upon the bishop and the bishop's world were blunted and turned back so that Jean Valjean had to confront his own life, his attitudes, his deeds. The person in need of forgiveness was Jean Valjean, and in this decisive moment of his life he found forgiveness and health. He forgot about the cruel world of the past and offered forgiveness to himself.

To offer forgiveness is the only way for one to have it, for in forgiveness, giving and receiving are the same.

ACCEPTANCE AND FORGIVENESS

The core of the process in psychotherapy relates to forgiveness. The unforgiving and the unforgiven are usually linked in the same patient. Recently, I saw a patient crying and wandering around a hospital psychiatry ward, repeating these words: "I will never see God. I hated my father. He died while I still hated him. And now I am beginning to hate my mother." This patient seemed to hear nothing but the message he kept repeating—a dirge of death. Healing for such a patient is achieved by the recognition". . . that only forgiveness heals an unforgiveness, and only an unforgiveness can possibly give rise to sickness of any kind" (*Psychotherapy,* 1976). This patient's therapy must be the passing of guilt, the obvious aim of forgiveness. Regardless of what the patient's past acts or attitudes have been, judgment will not help him.

The effective psychotherapist fully understands the meaning and relevance of the church's message of acceptance—"the doctrine of justification by grace through faith." This doctrine communicates to persons the good news that they who feel unworthy of being accepted by God can be certain that they are accepted. The pattern in psychotherapy of a nonjudging and nondirecting acceptance of the patient is illuminated by this profound Biblical insight.

Years ago, I read a story of a nurse's part in priestly absolution that I have remembered through the years. A young woman was brought into a hospital after she had been stabbed in a drunken brawl in a disreputable section of the city. All medical care possible was given her, but the case was hopeless. A nurse was asked to sit by the unconscious girl until death came. As the nurse sat looking at the coarse lines on a face so young, the girl opened her eyes and spoke: "I want you to tell me something and tell me straight. Do you think God cares about people like me? Do you think he could forgive anyone as bad as me?" The nurse was hesitant to reply until she had reached out to God for a kind of authorization and had also reached out toward the injured girl with a feeling of oneness with her. Then, knowing that she spoke in truth, she said: "I am telling you straight. God cares about you, and he forgives you." The girl gave a sigh of relief and slipped back into unconsciousness, and, as she died, the coarse lines disappeared from her face. Something momentous happened between God and that girl through the nurse (Horton, 1942).

Psychotherapists have many opportunities to be ministers of the grace of God. The psychotherapist may be an instrument of God's grace both in his work with the individual and with society. He may receive God's message and interpret it in a meaningful way for himself, for other individuals, and for society in general. Berdyaev (1960) emphasized God's way of working in our world:

> . . . God expresses Himself in the world through interaction with man, through meeting man, through man's answering his call, through the refraction of the divine principle in human freedom. Hence the extraordinary complexity of the religious life.

Through his empirical studies, the psychotherapist may give us a clearer understanding of the nature of man, of his dark side, and of his cry for redemption. Probably no professional group has taken more seriously the admonition of Carl Jung to wander with human heart through the world in order to study man in all the situations of life in which he could be involved. Jung encouraged those who wanted to learn how to doctor the sick with real knowledge of the human soul to visit mental and general hospitals, suburban pubs, gambling halls, brothels, places of business, revival meetings, and so on. When man is seen and studied in this context, one recognizes immediately that the relevance of the gospel is concerned not so much with teaching us how to solve such problems but with healing and regenerating the texture of the inner life of man.

Because of a nonjudgmental attitude, the psychotherapist may be accused of permissiveness. However, this permissiveness is often wrongly confused with moral indifference. In reality, this confusion has arisen because the psychotherapist has insisted that one's moral problem will be solved not by restricting and restraining the unknown impulses of one's depths but by allowing these to break through and to be used constructively. Man should accept his shadow or dark side and come to grips with it, or else he will become a victim of seriously disordered behavior. Mature morality is not a torturous and impossible obedience to any external standards, whether they are cultural and religious codes or personal ideals. True morality emerges through one's own nature, as one is made increasingly aware of one's own depths and of the extension of these depths beyond oneself.

The psychotherapist sees the meaning of neurosis as often having a relationship to a moral problem. The relationship here would exist in the sense that an individual gradually develops a rather rigid "conscious" moral image of himself, related to parental, religious, or cultural standards. Then, in the light of this image, he refuses to recognize the demands, impulses, or potentialities of his shadow or contradictory side. The refusal to recognize this other side and come to grips with it naturally leads to internal conflict or self-division, which constitutes the essence of neurosis. Paul understood this situation when he wrote: "For the good that I would I do not: but the evil which I would not, that I do" (Rom. 7:19).

Although those who work in the health professions may not have prepared for themselves a personal creed or statement of values, in spoken and unspoken ways, they attest daily to what they believe. It would be especially difficult for psychotherapists to hide their own value systems from their patients.

Because psychotherapy affects the values that determine life's choices, almost every kind of moral issue emerges during treatment. Although therapists may not dictate another's choice or stand aloof, they can explore with the patient the territory between these two extremes. They can raise relevant questions about which the patient has not thought, and they can supply pertinent information, permitting their own wisdom and insights to enter the picture. They participate in healing with what they themselves are, as well as with their studied arts. Their character emerges from both their knowledge and their behavior.

At no place does the saving power of charity become more apparent than it does in the process of psychotherapy. Often the patient, consciously or unconsciously, wants to be condemned. This may not be a healthy desire for moral restitution but an infantile seeking of punishment. Patients not infrequently tell startling stories of antisocial or immoral behavior, expecting to be preached at or given a moral beating. The refusal of the therapist to punish, reject, or condemn the patient often contributes to the patient's moral regeneration. This is the great paradox of effective therapy. The effective psychotherapist has always known that the deepest guilt feeling always comes from the message of grace and not from the proclamation of the law. In the world of the gospel, guilt is not dead weight but building material. In that context, the problem of guilt is the problem of love. One of the thieves who was crucified with Jesus did not indulge in lengthy self-accusations. He performed a simple act of love, and he was answered: "Today shalt thou be with me in paradise" (Luke 23:43). And of the sinful woman who kissed and anointed Jesus' feet, these words were spoken: "Her sins, which are many, are forgiven; for she loved much" (Luke 7:47). In both cases—the thief and the sinful woman—through the transcendence of love, there was no anxiety or struggle for self-assertion, for in the relatedness to Christ, the self was received as a gift of grace.

The essence of psychotherapy is to teach forgiveness and not condemnation, love and not anger or hate, inner growth and not self-destruction.

SELF-REGULATION

Great physician theologians such as Albert Schweitzer have re-emphasized for us the ancient truth that within each person there is a temple and a hospital: a temple where the Divine is firmly imprinted and a hospital where the forces that prevent illness or restore health are persistently active unless interfered with.

The body structure of human beings is composed of materials that, studied by themselves in isolation from their cellular environment, are characterized by the utmost inconstancy and instability. Yet the body has learned methods for maintaining constancy and steadiness in the presence of conditions that are threatening and profoundly disturbing. This ability of living beings to maintain their constancy under stress is called homeostasis.

One can go a step further and look at homeostasis from a psychological and spiritual point of view. Viktor Frankl (1959) has spoken to this issue when he postulates an inborn drive in the person that is called "the will to meaning." Thus, one strives to find purpose in one's own existence, to find a sense of mission that is uniquely one's own and that gives direction to one's life.

One should never underestimate the capacity of the human mind or body to renew itself, although it is often faced with what seem to be insurmountable odds. Most limits to this life force or regenerative power are self-imposed. The human breaks through or diminishes these self-limits by converting negative emotions to positive ones and by protecting and cherishing that natural drive toward homeostasis within him- or herself.

Where does physiological, psychological, and spiritual homeostasis come from? Since the earliest days of medical practice, physicians usually recognized that there was a power greater than themselves at work in the recovery of their patients. Whether this power is called God or nature or homeostasis is not important, for it is the recognition and acknowledgment of such a power that leads to the attitude of reverence in our work and in all of our relationships with human life. Since we need a fixed point of reference, a final cause and final answer by which to orient our human efforts, we can find it in this greater wisdom which controls the complex reactions of our psyche, soma, and soul.

It seems appropriate to go a step further and look at health enhancement as a form of self-regulation. For too long we have focused, in the health enterprise, on disorder and disease; we have spent too little time on the cultivation of simple rules and of a life-style that enhances our well-being. The brain harbors awesome restorative powers of self-regulation, unaided by outside chemical agents. When left alone to its symbols and when guided gently, it can do miraculous things. Like host resistance and immunologic competence, health is an active process, involving a participating client in a therapeutic contract with himself. As someone has said, the individual needs a pharmacopeia of personal and interpersonal skills to prevent his need for a pharmacopeia of pills. Dr. Joel Elkes (1978) of the Johns Hopkins School of Medicine has said that personal health needs, like the three Rs of Reading, Writing, and Arithmetic, the skills of another acronym, NERALT: Nutrition, Exercise, Relaxation, Awareness (including Body Awareness), and Listening before Talking. In aiding individuals in the way Dr. Elkes is suggesting, the health enterprise should broaden its focus in public health to include personal health and in behavioral science to include behavioral medicine (such as applied methods of personal health behavior).

While increasing our efforts toward the attainment or maintenance of positive health, the sick also need our concern and care. The sick person invariably asks, "Why am I sick?" Any one of three answers may be given. He may feel that an omnipotent deity has arbitrarily decreed this suffering to him as a form of punishment or in order that the sufferer may have a greater opportunity for spiritual growth through mortification on earth. At the other extreme, he may believe that his illness is the product of a complex evolutionary system in which he will be gradually eliminated by his own weaknesses. In this cosmology, the patient with his illness is like a short-necked giraffe or a porcupine without quills. It is more likely that the person will take a middle position between these two extremes. He may believe the universe to be governed by natural laws that seem to have been laid down for the conduct and evolution of life. At some level, his thinking may run along the following lines. Health consists in following these laws, and illness results from their infringement. Health is not thrust upon the individual but requires his active participation and is maintained by the constant practice of these rules, which are accessible if he seeks them. Although the health enterprise does participate in the discovery of these laws, it is the responsibility of the individual to follow them.

Probably, the shame and guilt that are so often felt by the patient arise from this uneasy sense of responsibility for his own illness. Although he may not be able to identify his own errors, he is dimly aware of them. As the philosophers have always stressed, "If a person will not study himself when well, he must when ill."

In studying any illness, one should always ask: (1) What does this illness mean for the individual in whom the signs and symptoms of disease reside? What are we being told about the person's emotional and spiritual condition? (2) What does this illness tell us about the family from which the sick individual comes? (3) What does this illness tell us about the community from which the sick individual comes? (4) What changes should take place in the individual, the family, and the community to help the patient regain and maintain health?

In the early twentieth century, it became widely accepted that stressful life circumstances, including interpersonal relationships, could be major factors in disease. Now, in the second half of the century, it becomes increasingly evident that such periods of stress for the person may have sweeping implications for illnesses of all kinds.

British physician Arthur Guirdham (1963) has suggested that for the relief of the chronic disorders from which we suffer we need another kind of doctor. He goes on to say that if the stress diseases are to be controlled, we must return to the conception of "the wise man." Such a person must have the knowledge and training of the doctor without his materialism, as well as the basic attributes of the priest without the paraphernalia of clericalism. Also, such a person will need the wisdom of the sage.

What, then, can we say today to sick persons? For healing to take place, medical knowledge and all that faith includes are needed. A combination must be made of what the doctor and the priest have to offer separately. When the doctor-priest is not available, it may be that patients will have to do the synchronizing, if health is to be achieved. In any event, patients have a mjaor responsibility for attaining within themselves such a state of balance that the natural forces of healing and renewal can predominate, whether or not they are fortunate enough to have the guidance of a doctor-priest.

In exploring the meaning of one's illness, perhaps the core problem is to repent, in the sense of rethinking one's way of life and one's goals and of clarifying what it is that gives life its meaning. Perhaps most often this sense of meaning is found in terms of certain persons, but it may be that dedication to certain aspects of creative production or work is central. Such was the situation with one young mother who had tuberculosis. She wondered why she should get well. Her realization of how much her young daughter needed her and was dependent on her gave the meaning to her life for which she was searching.

Another facet of repentance concerns the identifying of elements that are wasting life. Sometimes, it becomes essential to identify which elements of life are unrewarding or which are filled with dread. It will be necessary in some way to rid life of the elements that are bearing bitter fruit. This may be a sacrifice. It may mean giving up something to which a great deal of time and effort has been devoted without reward. It is often difficult to admit that in our choice of a way of life, a marriage partner, a certain vocation, or in moral decisions, we have been wrong. Or we may have to decide that we were not wrong—only lazy, stubborn, or misguided—and that proper application of ourselves would straighten out a disturbing and sickening situation.

Those for whom life has become so barren that there is no one or no thing to love must deliberately search for a love object. As a temporary, quick, and interim solution, one can use art objects, plants, pets, or other available nonhuman objects But this should never become a permanent solution to the exclusion of human love. Life is not fulfilled without human love, and the search for it must go on. Here, also, one can use temporary objects. Love and service for one's pastor, nurse, or fellow patients may be sustaining temporarily until a more appropriate and lasting relationship can be established. Love and service are linked, and through service, it is possible at times to find love. Love is the chief restorative power in the remaking of psychic health and wholeness. It is the only relationship invulnerable to the impositions of self that are the cause of much sickness. The cure for morbid self-consciousness is to divert the attention elsewhere, not by means of superficial distractions but by the investment of self in something other and better. A commitment can be made to certain work in one's family or community, in one's sickroom, or with certain acquaintances. This commitment can grow into a sustaining relationship. The effort to find love can tax one's ingenuity, but the knowledge that only thus can life be fulfilled will help in the search that must be made.

Thus, health is a state of the harmonious integration of the person within himself and within his society, nature, and the cosmos. Illness and suffering are indications that this harmony has been disrupted. The patient is considered, at least partly, responsible for this transgression; therefore, he must actively participate in the healing process.

CONCLUSION

It has been said that ideally psychotherapy is a series of holy encounters in which therapist and patient meet to bless each other and to receive the peace of God. In the therapeutic relationship as well as in other genuine relationships, the Spirit of God finds its temple. In psychotherapy, both patient and therapist share in the healing.

Something of the essence of a holy encounter can be found in an experience of Antoine de Saint-Exupery, a French aviator killed in World War II. In his *Wind, Sand and Stars* (1949), he tells how he and his copilot crashed in the Sahara Desert and how they wandered for five days without water and then were rescued. He describes their rescuer, and in his description is revealed how the patient and therapist must perceive one another if healing is to take place. Saint-Exupery addressed his words to their rescuer:

> You Bedouin of Libya who saved our lives, though you will dwell forever in my memory, yet I shall never be able to recapture your features. You are Humanity, and your face comes into my mind simply as man incarnate. You, our beloved fellowman, did not know who we might be, and yet you recognized us without fail. And I, in my turn, shall recognize you in the faces of all mankind. You came toward me in an aureole of charity and magnanimity bearing the gift of water. All my friends and all my enemies marched toward me in your person. It did not seem to be that you were rescuing me; rather did it seem that you were forgiving me. And I felt I had no enemy left in all the world.

The change from a model of illness to one of health rests in a large measure on the type of person selected as a student and on the training they receive in the art and science of medicine.

There are significant changes taking place in the current reappraisal of medical education. If approached with an open-minded attitude and a desire to improve the process of health care, it will greatly affect the future of medical care in the United States. If we are to encourage greater participation of the patient in his getting well and to recognize that treating the "whole" person requires an interdisciplinary approach, it means augmenting the present system of training physicians and other health care professionals. This will undoubtedly alter many concepts of the respective roles of physician and patient from those presently held.

Dr. Liebelt is a leader in the responsible changes taking place in medical education.

12

The Global Aspects of Health: Role Of Medical Education

ROBERT A. LIEBELT, PH.D., M.D.
VALORY MURRAY, M.A.

As the medical profession comes under closer and closer scrutiny in the media, physicians are increasingly subject to more criticism, less praise, and growing, sometimes contradictory, demands for change. The American public seems to be getting more and more uneasy about the entire state of medical affairs. Polls show that although individual Americans seem to be generally satisfied with their physicians and with the quality of their health care, as a group they are overwhelmingly dissatisfied with the health care delivery system. Everyone is unhappy about the ballooning costs of health care, and although physicians receive only about 8 percent of the total health dollar spent, the public seems to think they're overpaid.

Everyone is sobered by statistics indicating high death rates from heart disease, cancer, and a host of new diseases at the same time that both basic and clinical research proceed at an unprecedented rate of speed. Such statistics symbolize endless pain and suffering and suggest, too, that proportionately small amounts of useful knowledge and understanding are being gained from our research investments and/or that information transfer for the benefit of the patient is being seriously impeded.

The situation is not quite as bleak as it seems, however, because what we are actually presented with is a matter of "incomplete technology." The remarkable progress of sophisticated and costly scientific activity in medicine that is unique to the twentieth century and has been more prominent in the United States than in any other country has not been carried to completion. The history of scientific achievements in conquering polio exemplifies the process by which incomplete technology has become complete.

When polio first became widespread in this country, the costs of treating it and rehabilitating those afflicted with it were staggering. The costs of the research that ultimately led to the development of an effective polio vaccine were staggering as well. But once the right vaccine was discovered, technology allowed its mass production at a cost so low that from the perspective afforded today, the costs associated with early polio research seem almost inconsequential. When research into the causes and cures of such diseases as cancer, atherosclerosis, and muscular dystrophy has brought us to a point where technology can help to produce treatment phenomena as effective and inexpensive as polio vaccine, then the problem of incomplete technology will disappear with regard to these diseases, just as it did in the instance of polio.

In the meantime, the new public demands with which the profession of medicine is confronted seem almost overwhelming in their implications. There is, for example, a new public demand for de-emphasis on science in medicine in favor of a return to the art of medicine as it was practiced in the "good old days." Advocates of this change see medicine as currently dominated by excessively costly, cold, impersonal, disease-oriented doctors more interested in the disease or the fee than the patient. What they want instead is someone like Marcus Welby, M.D.—a man who warms his audiences more by his manner than by his scientific experience. This particular demand is evident, too, in the questions I hear in my role as charter dean of a new medical school: "What are you going to do about the social and physical problems of old people? Will your graduates be trained to deal with alcoholism and drug abuse? Will you concentrate on the effects of nutrition on health—and will you teach the public as well as your students? What are you doing to improve medical education about human sexuality?" I receive very few inquiries about the kinds of research we intend to conduct and whether we will seek the causes and cures for cancer, heart disease, emphysema, and other such potentially fatal diseases.

Somewhat paradoxically, in view of complaints about excessive scientific emphases in contemporary medicine, another new phenomenon with which medicine has had to cope is the manner in which new medical knowledge and technology has affected the public. Some people now seem to think that the miracles of modern medical science mean that all disease—and maybe even death, if cryogenics and cloning work out—can be conquered. Physicians seem to be thought of as near-gods (and some physicians behave as if they almost believe it).

These complicated attitudes have developed partly as the result of a new view of health care as a right rather than a privilege. As with other services to which Americans have become accustomed—for example, highway construction and maintenance, public transportation, and police and fire protection—we are beginning to take high-quality health care for granted and to expect its costs to be borne by somebody else.

In the midst of all the resultant clamor, medical educators now find themselves put on notice that a new definition of health is in the offing and needs to be incorporated in their curricula. Health is no longer the traditional "absence of disease": now, it implies emotional and spiritual well-being as well as physical well-being. Some even equate health with happiness and peace of mind and see the absence of these qualities as a determinant in the occurrence of the more familiar physical diseases. Those who espouse these ideas regard the majority of today's physicians as incapable of promulgating this broader concept of health and believe that other health professionals must assume the responsibility.

But the American public is also dissatisfied with medicine because of a feeling that established medical schools are either unwilling or unable to change their curricula so as to graduate physicians with genuinely broad educations. When people feel that they can't get responses to their health concerns from the health establishment, it is natural for them to turn to the mechanisms of government for help. Then we find federal financial aid to medical schools being linked to requirements for increasing class sizes, shortening curricula, and other, similar actions aimed at producing more physicians and differently oriented physicians in shorter periods of time. A kind of collective bargaining relationship has developed with the medical faculty and the practicing physicians on one side and the federal government on the other. For medicine, a profession with a tradition of one to one relationships, the new tensions between medical personnel and government has dramatic implications.

The medical profession is now addressing itself to the crucial issues suggested by society's new perceptions of health and the physician. Medical education is evolving in a manner responsive to the concerns of both the public and the profession at large. Medical educators realize that only through the instruments of education will future generations be assured that physicians graduating from our medical schools now will be able to provide the leadership necessary for assuring the best health care; however the definition of health care may be modified in the decades to come.

Change is, in fact, occurring; but, inevitably, it is happening slowly, and this pace is hard to accept in our turbulent time of the century. By its very nature, medicine requires of its practitioners a conservative temper. This is due in large part to the seriousness of its responsibilities. Physicians' concern for human life has bred in them a time-tested skepticism about hasty generalizations, a natural caution about experimentation with new therapeutic procedures, and an overall "go slow" attitude that can be frustrating and misleading to the public even while it works in the public's favor. It is understandable that the public believes that the profession of medicine is not changing, even though it is.

In order to gain a better understanding of how medicine and, in turn, medical education have evolved under these circumstances, a brief review of the historical perspective can be of value.

HISTORICAL ASPECTS OF MEDICINE

A hundred years ago, a knowledge of history helped some physicians and medical educators forecast the current health care crises. As today's medical personnel deal with these crises, a review of the sources of our difficulties seems in order, especially with regard to the ways that science and art have mingled in our profession.

The art of medicine began before history was written. As long as human beings have existed, someone has been responsible for dealing with human health problems, or with the "healing art."

Medicine as a science, however, is a relatively recent phenomenon, having had its beginning in the teachings of Galen in the second century after Christ. Plagued with error, the empirical dogma of Galen persisted for more than 1,400 years, its correction and improvement delayed by the fact that most medical theorists, like most philosophers, were busier attending to questions of man's place in the universe and his relationship to his maker than to questions involving man's physical functioning.

The systematic dissection of the human body by the anatomist Vesalius in the middle of the sixteenth century presented the first challenge to the long-standing traditions of Galen. The philosophical emphasis on self-exploration that began in the Renaissance helped bring the science of medicine into being and gave it such impetus to growth that the ensuing discoveries have gone beyond the wildest dreams of the early scientific explorers.

In the 1600s, the light microscope was invented, allowing exploration of the nature of fundamental tissues and recognition of the cell as the fundamental structural component; such explorations increased the knowledge of disease. Certain discoveries in chemistry and physics led to an understanding of the role of microorganisms in causing disease, and other discoveries laid the groundwork for the development, in the twentieth century, of the electron microscope, the differential centrifuge, the mass spectrograph, and the nuclear magnetic resonance spectrometer, all of which now permit man to explore disease at the molecular level.

In the late 1970s, we find ourselves in the midst of excitement about a new era of science featuring reductive analytic modes so precise and fruitful that belief abounds that identifying the tiniest parts of a phenomenon will lead to exact understanding of the whole phenomenon. It is no wonder that medicine has become so scientific. In fact, it would be a wonder if it hadn't!

But even among the strongest proponents of scientific medicine, there is a recognition that the tools of science are not sufficient to unravel all the mysteries of life. The nature of the complexities encountered in analytical, quantitative study of living matter suggests the operation of laws other than those currently known to physics and chemistry.

The long-held principle of linear causality (that is, A causes B which causes C, and so on) is being challenged by the concept of systems analysis, which posits that A, B, and C may influence each other in other sequences in order to produce different final effects.

Taking their cue from the finer and finer focusing of the traditional sciences, in the past few decades, the social sciences have begun to provide similarly finely detailed information about human interaction, primarily within family and community structures. Very recently, the findings of the traditional laboratory scientist and those of the social scientist who works outside the laboratory have begun to be seen as combined in a single continuum. This new continuum is now being offered as the basis for a new disease model in man in which disturbances at the molecular level are recognized as manifesting themselves eventually at several levels of organization: organelles–cells, tissues–organs, systems–individuals, families–communities.

In this setting the present vigorous, if not entirely precise, debate about holistic or (wholistic) medicine is occurring. In this debate, traditionalists assert that wholistic medicine has long been taught by medical educators who have sought to equip their students with the knowledge necessary for returning human bodies from states of molecular disarrangement to normal structural and functional harmony. Such instruction has entailed the disputed heavy emphasis on science and scientific techniques. Conflicting voices are now raised to assert that in medicine, at least, science has not borne out its promise. The new proponents of the "new and expanded" art of medicine suggest that the concept implies the existence of a vast store of knowledge and information that has not yet been fully identified, let alone put to use.

Certainly it is true that the art of medicine has not enjoyed the intensive exploration that has characterized the science of medicine. Experimentation going on now in parapsychology and the teleneural sciences is showing that certain physical and biological phenomena within the body, and most dramatically within the test tube, can be influenced by nontraditional healers. Carefully conducted experimentation is now being carried out in several highly reputable laboratories in the areas of parapsychology and teleneural sciences. These studies are demonstrating that certain individuals who have purported to have certain "healing powers" emanating from their body can indeed influence certain physical phenomena, such as deflection of atomic particles in a cloud chamber device, ionization of water that happened to be from the Lourdes Grotto, changes in the coronal pattern about the hands (recorded by Kirlian photography), and, more recently, activation of a chemically pure enzyme in a test tube. These "healing powers," so difficult to measure or account for, may be what patients have in mind when talking about "my doctor" and his or her ability to even make me feel better even without doing much.

But with all of this, it still seems that the issues behind the controversy between traditionalists and nontraditionalists are considerably more complicated than simple assertions about medicine as a science or as an art might suggest. It is possible that the virtues of medicine as an art have been viewed in a somewhat romantic fashion. It is important not to gloss over the fact that in the days before the explosion of the new scientific knowledge, physicians all too often sat by the bedside of feverish patients feeling like prisoners of their own ignorance, vastly frustrated in knowing that reassurance was the best they had to offer. Now, in this age of science, an exchange of telephone calls between patient, physician, and pharmacists produces rapid relief and, often, cures. Any physician who participates in such modern miracles of science will not be easily convinced that he should forego science in favor of increasing his artfulness. Art just doesn't seem to be that important to treatment.

HISTORICAL ASPECTS OF MEDICAL EDUCATION

"Three characteristic stages are to be discerned in the evolution of medical education" wrote Flexner (1910) in his report on medical education in the United States. The first and longest of these was the era of dogma, and its landmarks were Hippocrates (460–377 B.C.) and Galen (A.D. 130–200). The Galenic system took its place in the university, and facts had no chance pitted against the word of the master.

The second era was characterized by the dominance of empiric observation. Empiricists relied on experience and had little real opportunity to analyze, classify, or interpret phenomena. For the empiricist, the important thing was knowing that the extract of the foxglove plant could relieve "the dropsy," not understanding exactly how and why. Foxglove was used for several hundred years before its active agent digitalis was identified and its mechanism of action on the heart cell was reasonably well understood. Yet while the agent's nature and model of action were being elucidated, untold numbers of lives were being saved with this medication. Centuries later, a similar phenomenon occurred with antibiotics, which were used for the treatment of infectious diseases long before their principles of operation were completely understood.

The third era, of which we, today, are a part, is dominated by modern science, with its severely critical approach to experience. It is at once more skeptical and more assured than mere empiricism, and from its propensity for asking why, the process of reductionism has evolved.

The pressure of new knowledge has caused more and more young physicians to seek additional specialized training. Though such specialization increases their abilities, it also leads to greater restrictions on the numbers and types of patients they can see.

In the United States, in this third, scientific era of medical education, the master physician with his apprentice has moved from being the sole source of the training of future physicians through to the present situation, in which he has little or nothing to do with medical education.

It would appear that we may well be on the threshold of a fourth era in medical education, in which the characteristics of man that have been pondered over, argued over, and theorized about for centuries will be subjected to the sophisticated disciplines of modern science and technology as well as to the emerging psychosocial disciplines. In this new era, the definition of health as implicit in present medical school curricula will take on new connotations more expansive than the restrictive and simplistic definition of the absence of organic disease.

When America was being colonized, the only way to become a physician was to become attached to a practicing physician and, by observation, constant companionship, a little reading, and much imitation, learn the art of medical practice. This method was acceptable in the beginning because there were no medical schools. As the country's population grew and the demand for physicians increased, groups of physicians began to organize themselves into medical faculties, securing charters from state legislatures authorizing them to grant degrees. During the 1800s, 460 medical schools, many of them diploma mills, were chartered in the United States and Canada. The American system of medical education lacked structure and quality controls. It has been estimated that, in the early years of the nineteenth century, fewer than 10 percent of all American physicians were graduates of medical schools and more than 80 percent had never even attended lectures in a medical school.

Inevitably, serious American students sought out European universities for their medical education. The predominance of the scientific method in continental universities and the resultant predispositions of the returning graduates who had studied there led to the beginning of a reform movement led by the American Medical Association (AMA) that was to rock the entire field of medical education.

In 1846, concerned physicians with plans for improving their profession established the American Medical Association for the express purpose of advancing the standards of medical education. In 1891, the Association of American Medical Colleges was organized with a similar goal. But one of the most important events in the evolution of American medical education was the publication (in 1910) of a study now known simply as the Flexner report.

After scrutinizing 155 medical schools in the United States and Canada during a two-year period, the young nonmedical educator, Abraham Flexner, made public a report that was scathingly critical of many schools, suggested major improvement in others, and commended only a handful. It is estimated that the Flexner report was directly responsible for closing down twenty-nine medical schools in the four years following its appearance and still more schools in the subsequent four or five years when state licensing boards refused to allow students to sit for licensure examinations unless they had graduated from one of the sixty-six schools on a list approved by the Council of Medical Education of the AMA.

Clearly, the die was cast. The professional medical organizations had established themselves as effective arbiters of quality, and practitioners had developed a relationship with these organizations that persists into the present day. The majority of medical schools, attempting to meet the demands for higher standards and to provide an academic base for their educational program, formally affiliated themselves with American universities. New accreditation procedures and new opportunities for continued education were developed and accepted. A new type of physician entered into the private practice of medicine, sensitive to the importance of research and to the necessity of keeping abreast of new findings in the laboratory, even though his central interest might be patient care. In the course of about fifty years, the combined effect of all the factors fostering reform in American medical education resulted in such improvement that the medical teaching centers of the United States began to attract students from all over the world.

In the history of American medical education in the United States, the most illustrious practitioner of the art of medicine was the Canadian-born William Osler, who served for several years at the beginning of the present century as a faculty member at the Johns Hopkins University School of Medicine in Baltimore. Osler's years at Hopkins constituted a brief era in which the balance between the art of medicine and of science was satisfactory. Respect for the clinician reached a high point.

Osler had been trained in the British medical tradition in which bedside teaching and the development of superior clinical techniques were highly valued. His fame is due primarily to his profound and contagious concern for his patients and his students and to his broad knowledge of clinical medicine. The Oslerian tradition of medical education is still regarded with respect by the medical profession today. In the Oslerian tradition, the patients are viewed not simply as the carriers of disease but as whole individuals whose emotional and economic conditions require the physicians' attention as much as their physical condition.

Osler had been brought to Hopkins, paradoxically enough, by a leading proponent of the growing science of medicine, William Welch. Welch, Hopkins' first faculty member and for fifty years a major influence at the school, was a pathologist who had been trained in the Austro-Germanic tradition in which laboratory experimentation and its accompanying impersonality were predominant. Whatever the prejudices instilled in him by his own education, Welch recognized Osler's superior qualities and wanted him on the Hopkins' faculty. The few years during which Osler taught in Baltimore were important to the establishment of a creative tension and a standard of excellence that helped boost Hopkins into a predominant position of leadership. Medical schools all across the country adopted features of the Hopkins' model of medical education, including full time clinical faculty, emphasis on research, and bedside clinical teaching in an interesting, if somewhat disparate, blend of the British and Austro-Germanic methods of medical education.

Medical education was greatly affected by World War II which confronted physicians, medical researchers, and medical educators with urgent needs for improvements in the treatment of trauma, infectious disease, nutritional imbalances, and psychological problems. More and more funds for research were pumped by a worried government into medical schools and medical research institutes. The resultant improvements in diagnosis and treatment were truly phenomenal, and little public encouragement of government was necessary for the continued support, amounting to billions of federal dollars, of this biomedical research venture long after the ending of World War II.

But how had the postwar emphasis on research influenced medical education?

The postwar research push led to the development of a research-oriented academic who thought little about the system of teaching medicine as a healing art. Ironically, the intense interest in laboratory research distracted many faculty from guarding their curriculum time, and gradually a modest but nevertheless significant "opening up" of the curriculum occurred. First- and second-year students were actually seeing patients and could relate firsthand experience with disease processes to the concepts they were learning in the basic sciences instead of waiting, as usual, until the third year of medical school. The "lock-step" curriculum, in which every student is required to take exactly the same courses, was being modified.

The postwar surge of innovation and change brought students new opportunities, but it became something of a bane for them as well. Individual courses were retaining their autonomy as they incorporated more and more new knowledge, and insufficient effort was taken to help students see the connections between courses. For a time, students suffered from duplication of efforts, overlapping of material, and conflicting and confusing information about the same topic treated from different perspectives in several courses. The time was ripe for the development of an interdisciplinary approach to medical curriculum.

In the 1950s, the Western Reserve University School of Medicine (now known as Case Western Reserve) was to lead the way in meeting this new need. The school's leaders faced up very early to the problem of overspecialization and accepted the fact that vertical growth of various disciplines had led to a fragmented teaching program. They reshaped the curriculum so that each organ system could be presented and studied in an integrated manner. The method they developed has now been modified for adoption by many medical schools, both at home and abroad.

For the most part, the dramatic curriculum changes were confined to the basic sciences. In the clinical sciences, the Oslerian tradition proved more or less satisfactory. But although the efficacy of the bedside approach to learning clinical medicine has never been directly challenged, today's assumptions about the superiority of laboratory work in understanding disease threatens the development of the student's acquisition of personal clinical skills.

The bedside approach has been threatened, too, by the nature of the university teaching hospital. Like the Austro-Germanic clinics and institutes of the nineteenth century, university teaching hospitals today are characterized by the newest in thinking and technology. Students affiliated with them see only those patients most in need of the newest and most sophisticated diagnostic and therapeutic techniques.

It has been estimated that of a population of 500 people who become ill, about 250 will visit a doctor's office for treatment. Of these, perhaps fifty will be hospitalized in a community hospital, but only one will have a condition requiring care in a university teaching hospital or a tertiary care center. The patient population seen by the undergraduate medical student studying at one of these university teaching hospitals is composed, therefore, of those who have passed through a referral filter and who, by the time they are admitted to one of these many special beds, are probably considerably more knowledgeable about their illness than the neophyte medical student who confronts them. The student's experience will obviously be immensely different from the experience he or she would have had with nearly any of the 250 people who visited their doctors' offices and had no need to be hospitalized.

From this set of circumstances grows the observation that too many of today's medical graduates come out of school with an erroneous impression of "the real world of medicine" and are incapable of coping with the most common health problems in our society. And here, too, is the origin of the complaint that today's physicians are disease-oriented rather than patient-oriented.

There is often a lag time between the public's perception of the need for change and medical education's response. Response is slowed by several factors, including competition among courses for curriculum time, the orientations of influential faculty members, and the traditional concern of medicine for patient welfare, as noted earlier. But changes do occur in both the substance and the structure of undergraduate medical education. During World War II, an accelerated three-year medical program abruptly replaced the usual four-year sequence, and the need for more sophisticated medical procedures led to the ballooning growth of research and to an increasingly vigorous intellectual climate, fostering experimentation in the medical school classroom as well as in the laboratory.

EXPERIMENTATION IN MEDICAL EDUCATION

In new and developing American medical schools, two major forces now accelerate the movement of medical education away from the disease model and toward more of a community orientation. The first of these forces is public pressure, leading to the sorts of federal government pressure described in the first section of this chapter. The second force is the reduction of both public and private funds for the support of medical education. To start a new medical school along the Hopkins' model, including a university teaching hospital as well as a classroom and laboratory facility, now costs about $1.5 million for each student in the entering class—about $150 million for a class of a hundred students. This figure does not include the annual operating budget of the hospital. It is pretty clear why at least twenty-three of the medical schools founded since 1960 have been designed to depend on existing community hospitals and clinical resources for their clinical teaching programs.

In new and developing American medical schools, students are oriented to clinical medicine in the community teaching hospital, with its emphasis on ambulatory care and on common diseases and conditions, rather than in the university teaching hospital, with its complicated varieties of care for acute and episodic types of illness care. The linking of a medical student to a practicing community physician in many of the new schools helps to provide knowledge and appreciation of community health needs and preferences and affords the experience necessary for effectiveness.

What has been the effect of using existing facilities rather than mammoth teaching hospitals? Has the clamor for more patient-oriented physicians been silenced? No, it has not, partly because of the circular phenomenon that led to the disease orientation in the first place. As more and more full-time clinical faculty come from university teaching hospital educations to staff the new community-oriented medical schools, they bring with them their preferences for sophisticated techniques, their views that the really interesting patients appropriate for their attention are the ones with the most complicated conditions. Gradually, the new community-oriented medical schools affiliated with community hospitals evolve into the same kind of highly sophisticated operations existing in the university teaching hospitals with full complements of tertiary care capabilities.

But there are advantages as well as disadvantages to this evolution; the major advantage is the unquestionably improved quality of health care it brings with it. The major disadvantage, or course, is that as the patient population in the community hospital changes, the primary care physicians leave, and we are right back where we started in this modern era, with medical students coming to believe that they are more needed by the one than by the 250.

As medical educators, our dilemma is to find better ways of teaching those physicians who handle nearly 85 percent of the United States health care needs while maintaining the high academic standards of medical education in this country. One of several experiments in medical education designed to remedy these problems is currently in progress in northeastern Ohio at the Northeastern Ohio Universities of Medicine (NEOUCOM).

NEOUCOM's establishment was the result of the vigorous cooperation of legislators, community leaders, and university and hospital personnel from a seventeen-county region, all of whom recognized a need to relieve the region's physician shortage and improve the quality of health care while at the same time keeping down ballooning costs. They wanted to establish a school that would produce community physicians, physicians to whom the primary care of patients with common health problems would seem at least as attractive as tertiary care or scientific research or some other area in which concern for the health of the whole person is deemphasized.

The resources available to the planners of NEOUCOM were exceptionally rich: faculty, staff, and facilities of three major universities, ten large community hospitals, and two major tertiary care centers, none more than an hour's drive from the site chosen for the basic medical sciences campus. It was believed that the use of existing resources not only would be financially economical, but also would facilitate the development of settings in which students could interact with patients in an ambulatory care mode instead of with the very sick and often very frightened and excessively dependent patients found in the tertiary care modes of the university teaching hospitals where so many American medical students are educated. We suspect that it may well be a too-early and too-lengthy exposure to the exceptionally ill patient in the tertiary care setting which contributes to the tendency in many of today's physicians to consider their patients in terms of their maladies, as "chronic livers" or "bad hearts," for example, instead of as whole human beings whose minds and spirits require attention as surely as do their physical conditions. Patients in an ambulatory care setting are more likely than patients in a tertiary care setting to require their physicians to exercise interpersonal skills as adeptly as they display their textbook knowledge of disease and organic disorder, and this likelihood made ambulatory care facilities the most logical setting for much of our teaching to take place. The Ohio General Assembly provided $11.9 million for the building of Ambulatory Care Teaching Facilities at each of NEOUCOM's associated hospitals, bringing to a total of about $25 million the costs of building the necessary components of the new medical school. This is about $125 million less than the building of the traditionally designed university teaching hospital based medical school would have cost.

NEOUCOM's clinical faculty consists in part of hospital based physicians willing to add undergraduate teaching to their other responsibilities which, for many, include the teaching of medical residents as well as patient care and administration. However physicians in private practice in the community are also valuable educational resources and indeed, a major factor in the teaching program both at the graduate and undergraduate levels. It is felt that the practical experience of physicians engaged in caring for patients in community and community-hospital environments gives the physicians a sense of the value of the art of medicine that is missing in many of their more scientifically oriented counterparts, and that as these care givers direct and monitor the educational experiences of NEOUCOM's students, the sense of the art will inevitably be transmitted to the students.

AT NEOUCOM we try to help our students develop a comprehensive understanding and appreciation of medicine as a science. This process begins in the first two, premedical years of the six-year curriculum, which takes place at the consortium university campuses and continues through the third, extremely scientifically-oriented year at the Basic Medical Sciences campus in Rootstown where the students study anatomy, physiology, molecular pathobiology, neurobiology, and other subjects from a scientific point of view. The science of medicine is important in Years 4, 5, and 6 of the curriculum, too, but in these clinical years science is regarded as only one more, particularly valuable, source of support for the service of the whole human being rather than something whose practice should become an end in itself. We seek, that is, to reinforce in these years our students' intentions to become thoroughly educated physicians rather than scientists with medical degrees.

Just as we attempt to ensure a healthy balance in the teaching of the science and art of medicine at NEOUCOM, we also attempt to balance other curricular elements so as to encourage breadth in our students. The humanities program intended for the fall term of the student's sixth year of study is one example of this effort. In this term, principles of human development introduced much earlier in psychology and social studies courses and developed in the third year behavioral sciences program are emphasized and attention is focused on the crucial role that the physician's own mental and spiritual well-being plays in the practice of medicine. Students will be presented with more evidence of the need to develop and to be capable of sharing effective strategies for resolution of internal conflicts and with the testimonies of the arts to the needs of the human spirit for beauty and for truths that transcend particular times and particular places. We want the students to realize that their responsibilities to themselves are as multidimensional as their responsibilities to their patients and that fulfilling one set of responsibilities often depends to some degree on fulfilling the other. The humanities term is built on the assumption that we cannot expect our students to see the wholeness of their patients if they are not sufficiently conscious of the wholeness of themselves.

The objectives and design of the humanities term constitute only one of several unusual features of the NEOUCOM curriculum with its goal of producing practitioners of a more holistic kind of medicine. Other special features are the relative shortness of the time of academic study, six years instead of the usual eight; the opportunities our students have to return to their university campuses in the summers following Years 3 and 4 to take non-medical courses for credit toward the receipt of their baccalaureate degrees; the design of the Year 4 course called "Principles of Ambulatory Care" which offers our students exceptionally early contact with patients presenting a variety of common health care problems; and finally the consistent use of the "principle of revisitation," a pedagogic principle in which different perspectives on the same subject are presented in the context of several courses over the six year curriculum. In medicine where the expanding information base has led to the establishment of over eighty medical specialities and the lengthening of medical training to a dozen or more years, the revisitation principle promises to become increasingly important.

NEOUCOM's experiment in medical education retains the important features of a strong educational background in the basic medical sciences while strongly emphasizing early introduction to the practice of ambulatory care medicine in a setting where the family doctor's office becomes a classroom, and the family doctor becomes the teacher. The NEOUCOM plan teaches the student to learn at the bedside and offers the clinician as the role model. We hope that the simultaneous involvement of our students with the humanities and the social sciences while they experience doctor-patient interactions will help them to develop some of the humanistic traits—the arts—that medical graduates of the recent past are accused of lacking.

Most important, we hope the outcome of our experiment will be a group of physicians with broadly based understanding of community needs in the global aspects of health, the motivations and skills to implement appropriate programs addressing these needs, and a strong, well-founded appreciation and respect for themselves and for others as individuals.

THE FUTURE DIRECTION OF MEDICAL EDUCATION

Many of today's medical educators see the value in reexamining their present roles in the U.S. health picture, but their tasks are not easy ones. While maintaining their positions as guardians of the standards of excellence in biomedical research and clinical investigation, being sure that accreditation standards are met, and ensuring that the continually accumulating new medical knowledge is incorporated into the thinking of their students, they must also be sure that their own assumptions about and definitions of health are acceptable to the majority of the U.S. citizens. Clearly, the idea of health many now hold as fully involves psychological and spiritual well-being as it does the physical.

Experimentation must take into account the skills and contributions of other health professionals in various other settings than doctors' offices, clinics, and hospitals.

Efforts must be made to reduce the high degree of fragmentation in the health care domain. Medical educators can provide leadership in coordinating the vast array of health resources already existing in the community settings. Making use of the resources of universities, community health agencies, public health departments, local community hospitals, local industries, various types of community libraries, and so on will lead to the avoidance of costly duplication and to the improvement of the overall quality of the health and health care of the communities' people.

Medical educators need to focus more sharply on two target groups in particular: health professionals in service roles, and the general public. Both of these groups have growing interests in more and better access to health information. Providing such information will be beneficial in many ways, not the least of which will be more effective encounters between health professionals and their patients or clients.

The key concept in all of this is coordination, into which a check and balance system has been built. Linkage must be maintained between the problems, needs, and desires of the people in the community setting and the problems, needs, and desires of those in curricular settings. If the linkage is good enough, the education of physicians will inevitably improve producing doctors with better attitudes as well as excellent abilities to solve specific physical problems.

The sciences are central to a contemporary physician's effectiveness, and this fact will have to be recognized and given its due. Those chosen for admission to medical schools must be able to excel in their science courses. But we must put aside the mistaken notion that a talent for science and the capacity for feeling compassion are incompatible. The two can and do exist, perhaps especially in the students entering medical schools today. Students interviewed for admission today are quite different from those interviewed twenty years ago. Many of them seem more socially aware—more people-oriented—and more determined to maintain their own ideals of service to others than were their predecessors.

Perhaps more than anything else, medical educators must keep in mind the need to be sure that medical education does not destroy the attitudes and ideals these students of today bring with them.

The complexity of the health care system sometimes bewilders even the professional participant, much less the unschooled consumer of its services.

Where to go for help becomes increasingly more difficult to answer as layers of professionals are added to the system and as greater numbers of alternative resources become available.

Certainly, many of these services are a welcome addition to the health care program. By assisting an individual to re-establish the inner balance and harmony so basic to good health, such professional help can be an effective supplement to the basic medical attention that may be required.

Dr. Hayes addresses this problem and casts light on some practical steps one can take to select the best medical assistance in time of need.

13

Where Do You Go For Help?

DONALD M. HAYES, M.D.

The emphasis of this book is keeping yourself healthy and delaying the onset of disease. The keystone of such an effort is assuming personal responsbility for yourself. No one else can keep you healthy; you must be personally responsible.

Unfortunately, the prevailing attitude in our society is to the contrary, as is shown by the recently developed surgical procedure for bypassing occluded coronary arteries. The effort of the scientific community is directed toward finding such procedures, yet our lifestyles remain self-destructive. Thus, we merrily go on munching french fries, eating mayonnaise, and smoking cigarettes, secure in the knowledge that the surgeon can fix it all when the damage is done. Aside from the fact that the human body doesn't work that way, this entire approach is contrary to the idea of assuming responsibility for your own health.

Countless hours have been spent in a variety of settings trying to define health. Rather than deal with that particular intellectual exercise, I prefer to point out that health is neither finite nor static. One does not look at oneself and say, "Today, I have health." Instead, health is better seen as an ongoing process. Thus, the maintenance of health is a continuing job to be done by each of us. In order to be successful in this particular job, we must cultivate self-awareness, practice self-discipline, and develop the resources by which we can regulate our own daily rhythm, our diet, our sexual activity, and our pattern of activities in general.

However, despite all our best intentions and efforts, each of us, at some time or other, will reach a point when he or she must seek help related to health. Most often, this help will come from some segment of the health care system: physicians, nurses, pharmacists, and so on. This system has grown to such size and complexity that it is difficult for all but the most informed to know how to make their way through it.

Confronted by a backache, a fever, a swollen joint, or any number of other things, where do we turn? Do we go to the emergency room at the local hospital, to the family doctor, to the corner druggist, to a counselor, to a friend? The choices are increasingly numerous and confusing. This chapter is about such concerns. It is about how you can best use the health care system in your community, if and when you need it.

There are several levels of information and complexity which must be examined in dealing with this question. The first has to do with being sure that you possess accurate and adequate information about health and health-related matters. The next concerns those symptoms and circumstances that warrant the individual providing his or her own care—that is, medical self-care. In addition, there are several things that one can do on a regular basis that will be of great benefit in preventing illness severe enough to require health care.

Having considered these things, we can then look at when you should seek care and, having decided care is needed, at how to make your way through the health care system. Finally, it is necessary to look at the natural history of diseases in general so that we can reach an understanding of why this entire approach is reasonable and eminently sensible. Accordingly, as a conclusion, we must look squarely at the question; "Why bother?"

GETTING YOUR FACTS STRAIGHT

Some things about health are matters of *fact;* others are matters of opinion. There are almost as many opinions about health-related matters as there are different people. Unfortunately, some people hold these opinions so strongly that they come to regard them as facts, whether or not they have substantiating data. This is the first pitfall to avoid in being sure one's information is adequate.

The National Health Test, which was given on nationwide television in 1967, disclosed the level of our ignorance about some matters of fact rather than opinion. The results of this test showed that many Americans believed the following:

Bad breath means disease.

Daily bowel movements are essential for health.

A laxative is good for abdominal pain.

You feed a cold and starve a fever.

Alfalfa tea cures rheumatism.

Calories do not count.

Diabetes is caused by eating too many sweets.

Grape juice, honey, dried poke berries, carrot juice, and tomatoes are good for arthritis.

Olives, oysters, and raw eggs increase sexual potency.

In fact, none of these things is true. Although strongly held as opinions, there are no valid data to support any of them as facts. Certain of them, in fact, can be catastrophic if put into effect. For example, giving a laxative for abdominal pain can cause an already inflamed appendix to rupture, sometimes with lethal effect.

This list of responses makes one wonder just where we do get our information. Clearly, most of us recieve a lot of it from the media. And, of all the media, television is the most pervasive and the most influential. Part of the responsibility for the apalling misinformation shown above can be fixed here. For example, one commercial network TV channel was monitored by a panel of qualified medical experts during a 130-hour broadcast week. They determined that the content of programs and commercials was health-related about 7 percent of the time. Only 30 percent of this health time offered useful information. Seventy percent of the health material was inaccurate, misleading, or both.

Nonetheless, for many Americans, this is their major source of health information. There were ten times as many television messages urging the use of pills or other remedies as there were against drug use or abuse. Although some useful health information was offered, the major health problems, such as heart disease, cancer, stroke, accidents, hepatitis, maternal death, hunger, venereal disease, mental health, sex education, child care, lead poisoning, and family planning, were virtually ignored.

Without belaboring the point, there seems little question that the fund of knowledge of the average health care consumer is low. What then, must we do? How does one become an intelligent, responsible consumer? First, we must recognize that, to do this, one must be a skeptic about everything that is in print and everything that is heard, regardless of the source of the information. There are numerous "reputable" individuals in the health field, and there are also well-meaning neighbors and friends, who may disseminate inaccurate information. Because of this, there is a need to be critical and analytical. We must not accept statements at their face value but be ready to question anyone or any statement. This is not done with the purpose of being antagonistic but in order to assure the validity of the information, to clarify the remarks, and to better understand the purpose of the statements. As patients in the health care system, individuals must question matters of fees, diagnoses or treatments, surgery, and other such matters with their physicians, dentists, and other practitioners before decisions for action are made. People in possession of facts, not a melange of opinions, are in the best possible position to make correct and rational judgments about their own health.

MEDICAL SELF-CARE

Many common health problems are conditions that, if left alone, will clear by themselves. They are conditions which are more annoying than dangerous, more a bother than a threat. If we were left to our own devices, most of us could cope with such problems. However, we are not left alone. In fact, we are all but overwhelmed by expressions of concern and advice— from television and radio commercials, advertisements in newspapers and magazines, "news" stories of "miraculous" medical discoveries, and label claims on the products filling the shelves of drugstores and supermarkets. Not only do these things threaten our peace and our pocketbooks, but sometimes they also threaten our health.

The illnesses do not change much from year to year (although "hypoglycemia" is now more fashionable than "nerves" or "allergies"), and the remedies remain much the same. The old familiar "miracles" burst upon the drug advertising scene with regularity, only to fade with time and to be replaced by new ones. New deceptions are met by new regulations. Old fads are replaced by new ones. Fresh claims are cranked out to amaze and confuse the consumer.

The atmosphere produced by this constant media blitz is such that each of us is led to believe that he cannot survive even the most mundane illness without the benefit of one of these freshly marketed miracles. Because of this, many people now consult a physician for conditions that no one would have considered worthy of note a few decades ago. What is needed to combat this tendency is a move toward medical self-care for those conditions that are appropriate to it. Admittedly, there are medical conditions that are of such seriousness that a physician should be consulted immediately. But there are also many conditions for which people could care perfectly well by themselves. Patient self-care has the additional benefit of allowing physicians to direct their energies toward patients who truly need their services.

Dr. Keith Sehnert has developed an entire training program for patients encouraging self-care. This is described in detail in his book, *How to Be Your Own Doctor (Sometimes)* (1975). Another excellent reference to self-care is that by Vickery and Fries, entitled *Take Care of Yourself, A Consumer's Guide to Medical Care* (1976).

What are some of these conditions for which one can care? Probably the most common, and surely one from which the drug industries realize the greatest profit, is the common cold. We Americans spend over $735,000,000 per year on cold medicines. As a matter of fact (not opinion), there is no known treatment of value for this disease. Thus, the time-honored measures of fluids, rest, and, occasionally, aspirin, are as good as any treatment available. The disease will run its course in whatever manner it choses to anyway, and avoidance of toxicity from a variety of nostrums is more beneficial in the long run than the dubious advantages conferred by them. There are certain danger signals for which a physician should be consulted, and these can be learned quickly and easily from one of the books mentioned earlier.

Another condition for which self-care is as effective as physician care is influenza or "flu-like" syndromes. In virtually every instance of such illnesses, the best advice a physician can offer is to stay in bed, take plenty of fluids, use aspirin for pain relief, and wait for the symptoms to go away. Again, there are a few danger signals of which one should be aware.

Recent studies at a southwestern university showed that college students can be instructed in how to care for their own colds, influenza-like illnesses, minor gynecological complaints, and painful mentrual cramps. After being so instructed, these students actually experienced less disability and spent less time consulting physicians than their uninstructed peers. Surely the average person could learn the same material and apply it equally well to his or her own care.

"Well," you say, "If I accept as a 'given' that I can learn to care for my own minor illnesses, for what symptoms do I seek help?" This is a point well taken. The following is a list of conditions for which one should immediately call a physician:

Neuromuscular

Fainting, coma, lethargy, confusion.

Vertigo, dizziness.

Headache that is severe, unremitting, or accompanied by stiff neck.

Inability to see, flashes of light, severe eye pain, or sudden double vision.

Sudden weakness or paralysis of extremities.

Convulsions.

Change in mental state or speech.

Gastrointestinal

Inability to move bowels when previous bowel habits were normal.

Severe abdominal pain.

Blood in stool (indicated by bright red or black, tarry stool).

Inability to swallow.

Sudden, severe, profuse vomiting, with or without blood.

Profuse (not just one or two loose stools) diarrhea.

Genitourinary

Inability to pass urine.

Blood in urine.

Profuse vaginal bleeding.

Respiratory

Inability to breathe (due either to obstruction of the airway or a feeling as if you can't fill up the chest with air).

Marked coughing, severe sudden cough, with or without blood.

Cardiovascular

Chest pain.

Sudden rapid heart rate.

Irregular heart rate, particularly the onset of a very slow pulse.

Skin

Sudden onset of black-and-blue marks on skin.

Marked, profuse, and sudden sweating.

Blue (or any other color) discoloration of the skin.

Very high (over 103° in an adult) or very low (below 97.0° in an adult) temperature.

PREVENTIVE CARE

We have pointed out that it is important to avoid using the health care system unless it is needed. Failure to do so will bring us to all the consequences of using the system repetitively and inappropriately. Dr. Herbert Ratner (1965) described these consequences best when he said: "Modern man ends up a vitamin-taking, antacid-consuming, barbiturate-sedated, aspirin-alleviated, benzedrine-stimulated, psychosomatically-diseased, surgically-despoiled animal; nature's highest product turns out to be a fatigued, peptic ulcerated, tense, headachy, over-stimulated neurotic, tonsilless creature." Surely this is a portrait to which each of us would choose to give the lie.

In addition to learning our facts, learning self-care, and learning when to consult the system, what are some things we can do to avoid using the system? How can we actively promote our own health?

Mountains of opinion and voluminous anecdotal material attest to ways in which we can promote our health. But, in keeping with our earlier admonition, what are the facts?

The facts turn out to be amazingly simple. Dr. Lester Breslow and his associates (1972) have examined the health behaviors of large populations in sections of the United States for just such answers. What he found are seven simple rules for improving one's own health. What is most interesting is that these are things each of us was told by his grandmother or school-teacher. They are as follows:

1. Eat three well-balanced meals a day at regular times instead of snacking.
2. Eat an adequate breakfast every day.
3. Be sure to get *moderate* exercise (long walks, bicycle riding, swimming, gardening) two or three times weekly.
4. Sleep seven to eight hours regularly each night.
5. Avoid smoking any form of tobacco.
6. Maintain a moderate, steady weight.
7. Avoid alcohol or use in moderation only.

With regard to these simple practices, Dr. Breslow found that a forty-five year old man with none to three of these habits has a life expectancy of 21.6 years whereas one who has six to seven of them can look forward to 33.1 years. Looked at in another way, it was found that the health status of those with all seven good health practices is about the same as that of individuals thirty years younger who do not.

Surely these are behaviors for which each of us can strive without great difficulty. They do not require the intervention of anyone but the individual. If we are indeed going to assume the responsibility for our own state of health, I believe this is one of the foundation blocks of that effort.

HOW TO NEGOTIATE THE SYSTEM

The elements of the health services system are shown in Figure 13-1. Of course, particulars may vary from one community to another, but these are generally the pieces of the system as they can be identified. The largest and most essential element of any system is that for primary care. There are two essential parts of "primary care." First, it is the place where one goes to make first contact with the system when care is needed. Secondly, and equally important, it is the source of continuing care and of continuing contact with the system. The source of primary care has traditionally been the family doctor. However, in our present day system, it may be another kind of physician, such as an internist, a pediatrician, or even

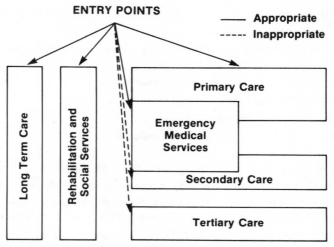

ENTRY POINTS

—— Appropriate

----- Inappropriate

Long Term Care

Rehabilitation and Social Services

Primary Care

Emergency Medical Services

Secondary Care

Tertiary Care

Figure 13–1 The Elements Of The Health Services System

a gynecologist. In many communities, the source of primary care is someone other than a physician. It may be a nurse, a school teacher, a clergyman, a counselor, or some other type of professional. In still other communities, the source of primary care may simply be someone recognized as having knowledge of healing and referral pathways but without any formal training.

In many large cities, individuals and families try to make the emergency system their source of primary care. The emergency system is an essential part of a comprehensive system for services. However, the element of continuity of care is missing here. You may take your child to the emergency room for an earache or a sore throat, and it will be treated adequately. However, if the treatment is unsuccessful or if the symptoms worsen and you must return, you find yourself faced by another person who has never seen your child before. Thus, each encounter in the emergency room is an entity in itself, and the staff must "start from scratch" in evaluating the medical condition each time. This is obviously not very efficient. Worse yet, in some cases it could be dangerous. Finally, it forces the staff of the emergency room to treat people for nonemergency illnesses to such an extent that they are often not able to attend to true emergencies when they arise.

Secondary care is comprised of the community hospital and the specialist physicians who practice there. Thus, if the same child with an earache mentioned above develops an infection that is resistant to treatment by the emergency room physician or the primary care physician, he will be referred to a specialist in diseases of the ears, nose, and throat. Whether the child is seen by this specialist in his office, in a clinic, or in the community hospital, this is still secondary care.

There are certain superspecialized procedures performed only in selected health centers, such as university or medical school complexes. Intensive cancer chemotherapy, transplant surgery, and reconstructive surgery are some of these. Generally, medical problems that cannot be dealt with at the level of secondary care are referred to a tertiary care facility. As one might imagine, this is a very small proportion of all those people who actually experience symptoms. The same child mentioned above might develop a brain abscess or meningitis from the resistant infection of his ear. In such an instance, this might warrant his referral to a university medical center, a tertiary care facility.

Although the elements of the health services system described so far bear a kind of orderly relationship to each other, the remaining two elements do not. Social-rehabilitative and long-term care are portions of the system that extend through primary, secondary, tertiary, and emergency activities. A program for social and rehabilitative services may be just as essential at one level as at another. Similarly, long-term care facilities such as nursing homes or convalescent centers function in the system without regard to the level of care being delivered.

In summary then, all of the elements described above constitute the health services system. A person may move from one portion of the system into another, may be in two portions at once, and may move about in it by referral, or on his or her own. Aside from the general lack of information about how to care for their own health needs, the other glaring deficit for most people is how best they can negotiate their way through the health services system. Many individuals consult practitioners inappropriately, as is shown in Figure 13–1. Many others do not consult one at all because of their uncertainty about where and how to enter the system. Being a responsible consumer includes obtaining knowledge about one's own health service system and how to best make one's way through it.

That is one of those things often spoken of but rarely done. "Exactly how does one learn about the system?" More pertinently, how does one make his or her way through it?

Step one is to identify and establish a relationship with a primary care physician. Admittedly, some communities offer no choice in this regard. Some have only one physician or one group of physicians. In such a case, it is still a good idea to go for a visit while one is feeling well and to establish a relationship with the only existing source of care. In other communities, there may be no physician, and the first contact person is another type of professional or nonprofessional. Generally, however, the choice of a primary care physician is open.

The next question to be addressed is: "What kind of doctor do I seek?" For an adult, the primary care provider is either a family physician or a general internist. In most rural communities, the family physician, either as a solo or group practitioner, delivers primary care. In many large urban areas, the internist is more prevalent as a primary care source. In any event, the more specialized a physician is, the less likely he or she is to be an appropriate source for one's primary care.

There are two qualities that every physician should have. One is competence, the other compassion. They are separate identifiable qualities, but, at the same time, they are indivisible. There can be no true competence without caring. A noncaring physician is indeed incompetent. A doctor who refuses to hear what his patients are saying, who is unable to inform or communicate ideas, who fails to express feeling or empathize with his patients, is an incompetent doctor.

Having determined what the essential qualities for your physician are, what about you? The ideal relationship between doctor and patient is a partnership. As with any potential partner, the personality, habits, and aspirations of this one must be known to you. After all, this partner may well hold your very life in his or her hands one day. In order to gain this knowledge, you must learn to be assertive, even though society has always rewarded you for revering the authority of the doctor. You must be at least as vigorous and forthright in this relationship as you would be in a good marriage or in some other productive partnership.

In this important relationship, exactly what will the primary care physician do for you? A good primary care physician will not allow your care to be fragmented by specialists. He will refer you to specialists for unusual problems beyond his ability or if you request a second opinion, which, on occasion, is appropriate. His function is as the integrator or coordinator in the team concept of medical care. Patients, too, are likely to fragment their care. They want a heart doctor, a kidney doctor, a thyroid doctor, and so on. All of these specialists reside in the secondary care tier of our health services system, and that represents an inappropriate entry point as shown in Figure 13–1.

What are some of the things you can find out about a doctor before going to him? Sometimes, his reputation in the community at large is worth exploring. Every successful physician has a host of patients who will testify to his or her greatness. Such testimony bears little relationship to reality and even less to his or her competence. On the other hand, consistent negative comments from a variety of sources should alert you to the possibility of problems.

Most public libraries have in their reference section a volume entitled the *Directory of Medical Specialists*. After acquiring the names of several potential physicians, they can be looked up in this volume. It will tell you where and when they went to medical school, where they took specialty training, and how much training they have had. It will also tell you whether they are board certified. If a physician has passed an examination given by the American Board of Internal Medicine or the American Board of Family Practice, he or she is more likely to be up-to-date and competent, although such certification does not guarantee competence.

Other factors of significance are whether he or she is on the staff of a teaching hospital, whether he or she is an attending physician at nursing homes or other institutions, and whether he or she is involved in civic activities in the community. Finally, before going to visit a physician, you should inquire about his or her fees. A doctor who refuses to discuss fees is displaying the worst kind of inability (or refusal) to communicate. It is well to bear in mind, too, that high fees do not necessarily guarantee superb quality of care.

Having looked at all of the factors mentioned above, you can only make your final judgment after a visit. There are many indicators of whether you have chosen the right partner for promoting your health. Some of these can be noted before you even meet the physician. If his office decor seems garish or inappropriate to you, look out! If you are compulsively neat and if his office is dirty and sloppy, you may clash. If his office nurse or receptionist is someone you feel you may have trouble with, make note of that.

Finally, before going in that office door, you must remind yourself of what Dr. Marvin Belsky calls "The Patient's Bill of Rights" (1975). In this listing, he points out that you, the patient, have the right to certain information, to access to your physician, to competence on his part, to confidentiality, to compassion, and to certain other items. If you feel, after meeting your physician, that you will have trouble getting these things, you would do well to look elsewhere.

Among the other attributes of an effective physician, he should be a positive role model for his patients. If you need support in avoidance of tobacco smoke and your doctor is a smoker, you have made the wrong choice. Likewise, if you are overweight and need help with that, walking into the office and meeting an obese physician should immediately tip you off that you are in the wrong place.

Another factor to be considered is the sex of your doctor. Ideally, this should not make a difference. However, if it makes a difference to you or to your physician, it should be dealt with. Some women feel more comfortable with a female gynecologist. Some men are uncomfortable being examined by a female. You should be aware of such feelings if you have them, and you should consider them in your choice of a primary care physician.

Less specific but more critical than any of these is a factor best described as "feelings." If your doctor "feels" right for you, that is most important of all. This is more than a simple like or dislike. It is a potential for open, honest communication based on mutual regard.

Finally, you should find out very specifically where your doctor stands with regard to health promotion and preventive care. If he or she is strictly an interventionist who sees no value in health promotion, you should turn elsewhere.

After all this, you should cultivate a continuing working relationship with your physician. He or she should become more than an entry point to the system for you. However, the creation of such a relationship requires an investment of time, a willingness to communicate, and some of the "personhood" of each party.

We have stressed the importance of the physician-patient relationship and the need for its development. Just exactly what things should be done within that relationship? Does that mean that you are supposed to return every twelve months or so for your "annual physical?" Not a bit of it! There is probably no greater waste of physician and patient effort in our country today than this anachronism. Instead, an individual who educates himself about symptoms that require attention, self-care for those that do not, and how to get attention when needed, can do some very specific things in partnership with the physician. A list of these follows:

Optimal Preventive Maintenance for Your Body

Infancy (birth to 1 year)

Tests for inherited metabolic diseases, congenital disorders.

Parent counseling about any of these found and about normal infant care.

3 to 4 visits to doctor for observation, immunizations, and parent counseling.

Preschool Child (1 to 5 years)

In the absence of disease, visit a doctor once at age 2 to 3 and once again prior to entering school for observation and counseling about nutrition; activity; vision; hearing; speech; dental health; accident prevention; and general physical, emotional, and social development.

For special high risk groups, blood tests for anemia, lead poisoning, and skin tests for tuberculosis.

School Child (6 to 11 years)

In the absence of disease, visit a doctor once at age 6 to 7 and again at age 9 to 10 for a complete physical-mental-behavioral examination with checks for obesity, vision and hearing defects, neuromuscular incoordination, learning disabilities, and completion of immunizations.

Health education and individual counseling concerning physical fitness, nutrition, exercise, accident prevention, sexual development, use of tobacco, alcohol, and other drugs.

Annual dental examination and cleaning.

Adolescent (12 to 17 years)

Health education and counseling in all of the above plus a course in sex, marriage, and family relations.

One visit to the doctor for the healthy adolescent (at about age 13) with special attention to psychosexual development and concerns related to puberty.

Ages 18 to 24

One complete physical examination with appropriate counseling before marriage.

Pregnancy

Childbearing education and counseling for both parents.

Ages 25 to 39

Instruction in self-examination.

Introduction of risk factors and appropriate counseling.

Ages 40 to 59

Complete physical examination every five years.

Ages 60 to 74

Complete physical examination every 2 years.

Counseling on problems on aging.

Ages 75 and over

Annual complete physical examination and influenza immunization.

Counseling on changes in body and in lifestyle.

Attention to these activities and others that may arise in different circumstances should afford you an excellent chance to maintain optimal health. This schedule will also disclose remediable conditions early enough to allow effective intervention in most cases. In fairness, I should point out that many physicians disagree with this approach. However, I must also point out that this proposed program is based on accurate data. Most individuals opposing it do so because of their own opinion, not because of contradictory data.

WHY BOTHER?

As we said earlier, the concluding section of this discussion should present a rationale for all of the foregoing. Of what value is accurate information in regard to one's health? How much good does it do to learn medical self-care? Why should we encourage good preventive health practices? What good does it do to know one's way through the health care system? In short, why bother?

The underlying rationale for all of the actions suggested can be best understood after examining Figure 13–2. It represents certain understandings that are common to all diseases in man.

First, it is important to understand that every disease has a developmental phase occurring before the actual phase of disease activity. The duration of this may be a few seconds or an entire lifetime. During this phase, the interaction of the host, that is, any person; the agent, for example, tuberculosis bacteria; and the environment produces the disease stimulus. The end of this developmental phase finds the stimulus poised, like a leopard in a tree, ready to pounce on the victim.

The attack of this stimulus on the host signals the onset of

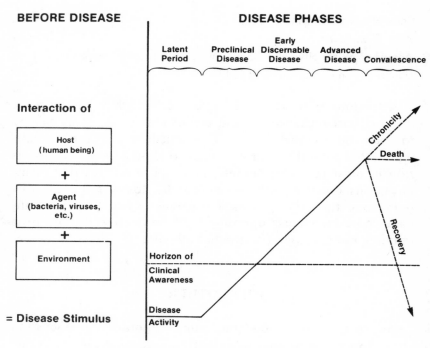

Figure 13-2 Natural History of Disease In Man

the second phase: active disease. The disease phase consists of five time segments: (1) preclinical, (2) early discernable, (3) advanced, (4) convalescent, and (5) resolution. The duration of each of these differs also, and each may last from seconds to years.

It should be noted that the line representing disease activity crosses another one labeled "Horizon of Clinical Awareness" at the phase of early discernable disease. This signifies that, even though the disease process is actively underway, it is not yet detectable at that time. Only when disease activity crosses that horizon can its presence be detected. Along with that, the higher the line of disease activity goes above the clinical horizon, the more severe and less reversible the disease becomes.

Now, with that picture of the natural history firmly in mind and reinforced by Figure 13-2, let us look at a specific disease, for example, tuberculosis. Here, the interaction of a human body, the tubercle bacillus, and an environment that may be cold, damp, or stressful produces the disease stimulus. The stimulus then acts on the body for a time, varying from days to years. This produces disease activity that may be detectable only by skin tests, since there are no symptoms. After the development of symptoms, such as fever, cough, or weight loss, the disease activity can be detected by a variety of means, including x-rays of the chest. Usually the detection of the presence of disease becomes progressively easier as disease activity increases. In the case of tuberculosis, time is important in another way. Treatment of a single case of advanced or chronic disease often costs several thousand dollars. If treated during an earlier phase, just after conversion of the skin test from negative to positive, treatment can be accomplished with about $1.50 worth of tablets. Even earlier on the time line, treatment or prevention costs still less. Elimination of any of the pre-disease factors can be achieved at virtually no cost. This is the point of the foregoing discussion. To prevent a disease before or just at the time of its outset costs pennies. To treat the same disease in an advanced stage costs thousands of dollars. To this monetary cost should be added the cost in time lost by the person and the cost in loss of body integrity.

There are other diseases, also easily preventable, to which this kind of analysis applies. Lung cancer, coronary artery disease, emphysema, and obesity are just a few of these. In each case, the disease can be prevented at virtually no cost by early intervention. Attention to lifestyle, diet, smoking behavior, and such items can accomplish this. On the other hand, allowing such diseases to progress forces us into a position where inadequate and expensive treatment may be the best option we have.

Thus the answer to "Why bother?" becomes obvious. By bothering early enough, we can avoid some diseases entirely. Even after the establishment of disease, a certain amount of bother minimizes the difficulty and expense of treatment, decreases disability, and eliminates mortality.

Perhaps the best illustration of the trials of medical care is a verbal one from Oliver Wendell Holmes (1976): "There is nothing men will not do, there is nothing they have not done to recover their health and save their lives. They have submitted to being half-drowned in water, and half-choked with gases, to being buried up to their chins in earth, to being scarred with hot irons like galley slaves, to being crimped with knives like codfish, to have needles thrust into their flesh, and bonfires kindled in their skins, to swallow all sorts of abominations, and pay for all this, as if to be singed and scalded were a costly privilege, as if blistering were a blessing and leeches a luxury."

Note that this picture is couched in phrases describing things we have allowed someone else to do to us. Isn't it a shame that we are not willing to assume responsibility for what we do to ourselves and avoid much of that? Each day, each of us moves inexorably up the line of some disease activity toward irreversibility, disability, or death. By attention to our own health *now,* that progression could be reversed or arrested.

14

The Future Starts Now

ELLIOTT M. GOLDWAG, Ph.D.

The aim of this book has been to share with the reader better ways of dealing with disease, of understanding its basic causes, and of establishing the foundations for true health. I believe that the path to unified medicine is ultimately through spiritual psychotherapy.

The key concept is that disease is the consequence of how we perceive stress and that we can change those forces within us that make us more susceptible to the stressful pressures that often accompany change. By adopting the attitude that stress can be neutralized or used positively, through the disciplines described in this book, we need not ever get seriously or chronically ill.

One of the major implications of the findings and perceptions offered in this book is that the problems of our mind and the problems of our body emanate from an alienation of the spirit, or soul, of man. We can learn to know our souls again through some of the methods and exercises described by our many authors. The issue comes down to our relationship with God, Who dwells in our inner self. By getting to know ourselves ever more deeply, ever more compassionately, we come to know God.

We are not really talking about old-time emotional spirituality. Nor are we resurrecting the hair-splitting mentality of historical doctrines. What we are seeing is the emergence of a new spiritually oriented science that has as its goal the restoration of harmony between God, man, and nature. The combination of concepts is so new, however, that we are required to change our thinking about science and spirit. We need, once more, to begin to see science and spirit as one. This, too, is the aim of this book.

Let us carefully try to discuss what seems to be happening today and where we might be going. In a practical sense, through this explosion in thought and its power for change, we can expect truly a new age for mankind.

First of all, it is my belief that the world is already passing through a tremendous number of changes. These changes range from a new alignment of global political forces to disruptions in our social and economic systems. The details and framework can be found on the front page of any newspaper. Alvin Toffler, in his important book, *Future Shock* (1970), gave us a vivid description of what society is now experiencing. The re-evaluations are certain to bring enormous changes in our individual lives, and we are going to have to learn to handle those changes and the possible stresses they produce. That necessity will form the basis of a new, scientifically based approach to medicine that can help the stressed individual transform his own set of spiritual values, his own realities of what life is about, in a time when humanity will need to learn to share more and to live together more harmoniously.

The first concept to understand is that the body is an energy system. In fact, it is made up of many energy systems, from the transformation of food into muscle movement, which biochemists study, to the production of energy fields around the body, which science is only now beginning to detect. It is all one system of varying levels of energy flow and vibratory rates. Many of these energy states cannot be measured precisely today. But some states have already been measured. One of the most significant discoveries in medicine and biology, it seems to me, has been sadly overlooked. For over thirty years, Dr. Harold Saxton Burr, a professor of anatomy at Yale University Medical School, performed thousands of experiments that confirmed (with precise measurements) the existence of what he called "fields of life" in all forms of life (Burr, 1972). All living forms from trees to man, Dr. Burr and his associates learned, are moulded and controlled by electromagnetic fields (L-fields) that keep living things in their shape and to which our bodies and minds respond and, in turn, also influence. Further, mind or thoughts produce *measurable electrical changes* in these L-fields. Think of the extraordinary tools tomorrow's physicians will have for determining health status.

What scientists are beginning to find is the immense power of thought to alter the body's internal system and its related energy fields. Joy, it is being found, generates a physical field. Despondency generates its own field. These fields, some say, can now be seen only by certain individuals gifted with the ability to see what are called "auras," frequencies of energy picked up by the aura reader's ability to fine-tune his mind and thus become a sensitive biological antenna. We are told that all people possess this undeveloped ability.

But my aim is not to make a scientific case for the existence of the aura or to find reasons why some individuals can read these energy fields. The point is to underscore that thought is the originator of those fields. Thought patterns conspire to imprison us in despondency. But spiritually based thought patterns can raise us to feelings of confidence and unity.

All the authors appearing in this book can be seen both as prototype researchers and as practitioners of a unified medicine. These practitioners remind us to be more whole, more loving, less attached to those things that we identify with security, and, in the spirit of science, more observant of relevant subtleties of mind and body. They also are all conscious of their spiritual selves. Their scientific work is motivated by spirituality and by love. Science, they are showing, is moving us ever closer to the reality of God, and the most obvious avenue seems to be through health and medicine.

One example of current research on the power of thought opening the way to a unified medicine is in the field of bio-feedback research. Biofeedback is demonstrating clearly the skills within each of us to control body functions in ways never before thought possible. Another is Kirlian photography, which presents physical evidence of energy fields, apart from the apparent phenomenon of auras. Biorhythm and chrono-biology studies are teaching us about the exquisitely subtle forces that generate in us cyclical patterns of emotional, intel-lectual, and physiological states that will certainly be used to establish a wiser system of therapeutics. And we are finding that our bodies and minds respond distinctively to electromagnetic fields. All this work bespeaks a sensitivity of that body-mind combination that today's science and medicine are only be-ginning to discover. Thoughts that arise through our spiritual awareness however, is the force that unites all men. Such thoughts are the most intense and powerful because they seek God.

In his book, *Psychiatry and Mysticism* (1975), University of Miami researcher and physician, Stanley Dean, says, "Thought is a form of energy; it has universal field properties which, like gravitational and magnetic fields, are amenable to scientific research. Thought fields can interact, traverse space, and pene-trate matter more or less instantaneously. Thought fields survive death and are analogous to soul and spirit. Thought fields are eternal; hence, past existence (reincarnation) is as valid a concept as future immortality."

What exists physically exists first in thought and feeling. If we do not like the kinds of experiences we are having, we need to change the nature of our thoughts and expectations. Then our behavior will change. There needs to be an alteration in the kinds of messages our thoughts are sending to our bodies, to our friends, and to our associates. The key to better health, to more productive interpersonal relations, rests within us and our ability to exercise and direct the nature, shape, and form of our thoughts along generous and spiritual lines.

Dr. Andrew Weil, author of *The Natural Mind* (1972), says, "The only limits we encounter in the world around us are those we first create in our imagination."

There has always been significant debate around the field of parapsychology, which is really the study of unusual forms of human energy. We already know how thought and perception can produce changes in our body chemistry. Researchers led by Dr. Robert Becker (1972) at Veteran's Administration Hospital in Syracuse, New York, are demonstrating the unusual capacity of direct current electricity to accelerate the healing of wounded tissue and the mending of broken bones. And at a meeting of orthopedic surgeons last year, Dr. C. Andrew Bassett reported on the treatment of bone fractures that resisted healing. Using a form of electromagnetic therapy that effected tissue changes, he indicated that of the 200 cases treated, 85 percent successfully responded to this form of therapy. Some beginning scientific work has been done to understand the energy fields generated by the hands of healers through their effects on enzyme activity (Smith 1975).

The growth of psychedelic research, Gestalt psychotherapy, bioenergetics, the human potential movement, and encounter groups has injected many added dimensions into the understanding of consciousness. And laboratory techniques for inducing altered states of consciousness are enabling one to see the interesting similarity between reports of ancient religious and mystical schools and current reports of transcendent experience.

Students of human development know that the search for meaning seems to be most often satisfied when people go through some extraordinary event in their lives that has a marked change on their consciousness, particularly in their beliefs about who they are and what they are doing here. Those who manage to get in touch with those inner spaces seem to have achieved a greater degree of freedom in their lives, a greater sense of inner peace, and a more satisfying style of life.

What we are saying is that self-direction, or regulation, is intimately related to our beliefs about who we, as persons, are. What our self-identity is will determine how we will re-create our biology and our environment.

"For me," says Dr. John Lilly (1977), a scientist famous for his explorations of the deep self and inner realities, "a most important lesson of the past several years of my life has been the realization that each of us is totally responsible for whatever is going on in our lives. . . . Wherever I am and whatever is occurring in my life, I am responsible for being there, and I am responsible for changing it if it isn't satisfactory."

Taking responsibility without selfishness or without indifference to the feelings of others requires dedicated work. For frequently we may be misunderstood by others as we seek a fuller existence for ourselves. As we move on the path toward inner knowledge and development, we very often may be misunderstood in our attempts to change relationships that we may find limiting to our own development.

Growth, in other words, takes courage, because we may be lonely from time to time as we move toward a deeper understanding of freedom and love. The loneliness stems from the process of giving up old ideas that were symbols of security. It is a process of clearing out the viruses of our mind—those habits of thought that have not been loving or generous. We may upset ties that may be important. But on the other hand, every moment is a new period in our lives. As quickly as an old relationship is abandoned, it can be re-established in a better state than it was in before.

The point to be made again and again is that the predominant path is toward self-reliance, with the knowledge that we are responsible for our thoughts, our beliefs, and our illnesses and that we can change.

The more we are taught to rely on ouside explanations and solutions for our health problems, the less confidence we have in our own innate abilities to heal. If the thought processes that produced the need for illness persist (whether one takes vitamins or gains temporary relief from pills, or visits his physician, or has surgery), the illness will return in another form. What is the point of curing symptoms when another symptom is always there to be chosen?

If we believe we are overweight, it is not the eating that produces the overweight. It is the belief that we are fat that produces the eating. This is because our physicial "set" of obesity is programmed by our self-image of who and what we are. Dieting reinforces the condition because we so deeply believe in our overweight condition.

One who truly seeks truth from within, in his own personal experience with Nature, the Life Force, or God, will always find himself establishing connections, common denominators, and a closer relationship with mankind. As one psychologist, Ira Progoff (1975), suggested:

> . . . It is as though each of us is a well. We are engaged in entering that well, which is the well of our life, and in reaching as deeply into its sources as we can. . . .
>
> We each go down individually into the well of our life. The well of each personal existence is separate and distinct from every other. Each individual must therefore go down his own well, and not the well of someone else's life. We find, however, that when, as individuals, we have gone very far down into the well of our life, we come to an underground stream that is the source of all the wells. While the wells of our personal existence are each separate from every other, there are no separations here. There are no walls or dividers in the underground stream. We are all connected here in the unitary continuum of being. . . .
>
> Just as we cannot live someone else's life, so we cannot go through someone else's well to reach the underground stream. We each must go through our own personal existence, but when we have gone deeply enough we find that we have gone *through our personal life beyond our personal life.* This is the transpersonal connection which we experience in the underground stream. . . .

The process of reaching our deepest sources, of revitalizing ourselves by connecting with the larger unity, and of using this replenished energy to deal with the outer events of our lives, is a continuous one.

What practical effect will these ideas have on the health system? We have already seen how such probings, such efforts to establish more positive realities can produce a constant state of health. But what of the system at large?

We are witnessing the re-unification of psychology and biology as well as a new flowering of spirituality with respect to the healing process. They are slowly coming together as one, and medicine will eventually take full institutional cognizance of this phenomenon. It is true that some medical students may enter the profession for its financial rewards. But on the whole, knowing that medical education is expensive and exhausting, young people decide to become doctors out of an idealism that reaches back to Hippocrates. It is still a spiritual thrill to receive the degree, Doctor of Medicine. Curricula are changing, along the lines described by Dr. Liebelt in Chapter 12. The science of medicine and the art of medicine will once again become equal partners.

Medical students today are overwhelmed with extraordinary amounts of information to learn and memorize, all for the purpose of educating themselves in the discipline of scientific medicine. This sort of education may be suitable for training research physicians and other specialists to intervene in acute situations, to perform surgery, and to deal with other emergency problems, so they are an integral and essential branch of medicine.

But perhaps what we need now is a type of training in the same medical schools for students who would be educated heavily in the fields of behavioral medicine, preventive medicine, and psychosomatic medicine, where the emphasis would be on the role of the mind in disease and illness. These doctors would be called doctors of health. These physicians would intervene in illness states through being teachers and guides to their patients in the joint process of exploring life-styles and other influences. There would be more concentration on developing the intuitive talents in such physicians; that is, those intangible human qualities that were characteristic of the great humanistic physicians who were loved by their patients. This intuitional talent, or clinical sense, is spiritual quality promoting healing just by its presence. A healer—a true healer—is a guide in developing our own sense of autonomy, which is really a rediscovery of the love that is in us all.

Dr. Hilliard Jason (1977), director of faculty development of the Association of American Medical Colleges, gave his perceptions of holistic medical training in a symposium given in 1977:

> What we want is people who are vigorously alert to their own limitations and respectful of the strength of others, and yet the characteristics of a great deal of what goes on in the educational process focuses almost exclusively on the issue of being right, rather than acknowledging all ways in which one is likely to be wrong. Contrary to our long standing reports and assertions, a great deal of what happens in education, as in health care, is self-serving; it is for the good of the provider, whether of education or of health care, rather than for the good of those being served. The image of education, I think, is nicely summarized in that ancient saying that, "If you give me a fish, I can eat for a day. If you help me learn how to fish, I can eat for a lifetime."
>
> The way we keep medicine and education mystified so that people don't learn to do their own fishing and managing their own affairs keeps a lot of teachers and doctors feeling that they have job security, but it doesn't provide the kind of individual development that folks need. The effect of all this is the difference between a relationship that is controlling and one that is liberating or strengthening to the person or the group that is the receiver of care or education.

And Dr. William F. Maloney (1977), Director of Education Service in the Department of Medicine and Surgery at the Veteran's Administration, calls for the need of physicians to develop considerable self-understanding in their training. Emotional growth comes with years of experience, years of simply living through crises. Therefore, we cannot expect the young physician to attain the necessary emotional growth by his or her mere presence in medical school. There is a great need to develop in the young physician the basis for self-acceptance and self-understanding. "Without that," Dr. Maloney says, "how can one help others attain these? Isn't that the basis of being one's own physician?"

"I have to first know me before I can really know anyone else," says Dr. Hiram Curry (1977), Director of Family Practice at the Medical University of South Carolina. "I have to be comfortable with me, imperfect, fallible me, before I can build a satisfactory relationship with imperfect, fallible others. I have to be able to tolerate these imperfections in me before I can tolerate a non-compliant patient and what that means."

These new approaches to the development of the physician— that is, the healer—have huge implications for the treatment of patients in the future. Rather than developing a dependency relationship between the patient and ourselves, the treatment setting turns into a process of two people working out between them the possible causes for discomfort. Then together, as equals, they work out possible solutions.

We, as patients, assume our responsibility as participants in this process and as contributors to our dis-ease or discomfort. The physician assumes the role of a teacher who, having spent a great deal of time training himself, can recommend temporary interventions to relieve pain and remind us of dissonances in our lifestyles that prepared the soil for the establishment of our illnesses.

Because the doctor is continuing to work on his own problems—with the help of his own set of "teachers"—he reaches heightened sensitivities that allow him greater empathy with his patient. Empathy is the essence of the healer. Without it, we can be of little help to others. It comes from compassion for oneself and from the willingness to examine and root out the ideas that alienate us from God, ourselves, and others.

It is true that many of us may find it difficult to give up old ideas and that we would rather function in the old medical model. But as scientists or professionals, we can no longer be content to live the schizophrenic life of being a reductionist in our office work and a whole being in our personal life or as Karl Pribram (1978), the brilliant brain researcher suggests, seeing "with a telescope in one eye and a microscope in the other." It is no wonder that many professionals suffer from the same conflicts that beset their patients. It is typical of what C. G. Jung called, "split consciousness," so characteristic of the mental disorder of our day. All of us are in need of healing.

As I write this chapter, I must continually remind myself of my own processes of growth. Although I can talk about the meaning of the new medicine, I acknowledge my own continuing susceptibility to disease if I permit the misuse of my thought energies. The message is, of course, that we must continually work to diminish the programming that led us to our state of unease. We are always susceptible to sneak attacks of stress. Life is complicated, but it needn't be as overwhelming as it is to so many, so that they must resort to tranquilizers, barbiturates, and antidepressants.

We are all healers, whatever our occupation. As we develop, we will learn to heal relationships with those from whom we are alienated. The message has been repeated to us over and over by great philosophers, religious leaders, inventors, and contributors to the advancement of scientific thought. Now we are seeing the need for mutual healing—of ourselves, of our planet—as a practical necessity.

What we see is what we believe we are. We have the choice of seeing the world as hateful and competitive or as beautiful and basically unified. We make our reality. It is really a matter of the kind of reality we want to choose, the kind of personal world in which we want to live. We can always decide that we've had enough of negative thinking and choose new thoughts that are better substitutes for old ones.

The alcoholic who joins Alcoholics Anonymous, finally gives up drinking, and sees himself in another way has exercised a choice. He gave up what he thought he needed and chose a better way, a spiritual way, for Alcoholics Anonymous is clearly spiritual psychotherapy.

All of us may need to reach some point of "bottoming out" when we decide we have had enough suffering and choose to renew ourselves. In doing so, we always change some aspect of our beliefs about what we thought was so, finding it was not.

Most often our belief system becomes a self-fulfilling prophecy. If I believe I will fail on an exam because I haven't studied as much as I believe I should have, then the likelihood is that I will fail. The failure has nothing much to do with whether or not I have studied, but it results because I *believe* that failure is inevitable because of insufficient study.

The expansion of personal consciousness we are describing here will lead to a need to reconsider the kinds of institutions structured to serve people who are ill. One needs to distinguish between places where acute intervention will be necessary and places ,where chronic conditions will be treated. Our hospital system is second to none for meeting acute care needs. But most of our hospitals operate on the disease model and are not ideal environments for recovery. It appears to me that we need an alternative to hospitals or illness centers.

Health centers or wellness clinics, where the atmosphere, staff, surroundings, and energies are devoted to health and to the encouragement of such thought, produce an environment totally different from the disease centers. They would be devoted to preventing illness and to counseling those who are recovering from ailments.

Such wellness centers, described in Appendix A, would be staffed by teams of health professionals who have reached points in their own professional careers where they are disenchanted with the inadequacies of our present system and have sought change by working on their own personal growth. Such personnel have usually reached some level where they recognize that the process of healing can be helped in a variety of ways, by a variety of professionals, and that the basis of all healing is the love and care expressed by one human being for another.

In such an environment, with an encouraging kind of atmosphere, with a variety of instruction and guidance available, and with the main focus on helping people to help themselves, personal growth of personnel and clients becomes a mutually rewarding and supportive experience.

Such health centers would be organized to use teams of helpers such as doctors, nurses, social workers, psychologists, and pastoral counselors. Each health task would be performed by the staff member most able and qualified to do it. Such centers would be ideal places where a wider use of nonmedical professional helpers could be implemented. Patients would thus be able to participate more in the management and treatment of their everyday illnesses.

Such health centers can include teaching and research in fields such as family practice, so neglected today. Because of its emphasis on primary care, I would visualize medical schools developing affiliations with wellness centers, just as they do with hospitals. There seems to be a need for closer relationships among primary care, health-focused physicians, and academic medicine. The nucleus for such centers has already begun in various parts of the country.

Such a center would encourage people searching for a better way to find the means by which their consciousness can grow and to begin to look within themselves for the answers in their lives. As a learning center, this environment can help people recognize that there are reliable guides to action from increased self-awareness. We may call such a guide an Internal Teacher, God, or any other name—it is the recognition that there is a higher meaning—a spiritual force, which guides our destiny and that of the Universe—that brings us into a group consciousness, causing a unifying experience rather than segregation.

Throughout this book, the reader has no doubt sensed a common thread—the importance, in every aspect of our lives, of developing the right brain consciousness of becoming in touch with our inner realities, or our spiritual, intuitional selves. I have placed emphasis on the choice all of us have at any given moment of our lives to choose one thought or another that will guide our actions, our behavior, and our physical condition.

You may ask how it is possible to change thoughts to bring oneself into this awareness, to overcome all of the past programmed hierarchies of thought forms that have caused us to act and react in our lives. For some, it takes years of some type of psychotherapy to begin to change or to see things in a different light.

I believe that the lengthy process of psychotherapy can be

shortened by the awareness that the past does not exist any-more in the present moment and that by dwelling on the past one only continues to examine every detail in a reductionist fashion, fragmenting oneself into smaller pieces of individual experiences that can cause one to lose sight of the primary objective. Although certain traumatic events can have special meaning and purpose in our belief system and need to be recognized, the belief system itself needs to be the primary focus of attention to help us become conscious of who we really are, not who we have thought we are.

I do not wish to be glib about the process of change. There are those who have experienced change in short periods of time, when they were willing to forget an old idea about themselves and accept a new, more satisfying life. But, usually, it does require regular practice in order to undo years of encrusted habits. Science writer, Itzhak Bentov, suggests that there are three ways change happens to people:

1. Change that is slow and easy to handle.
2. Change that we push ourselves into through meditation or some other self-growth process.
3. Change that is unsolicited and sudden.

Change of the latter two varieties is happening to many people I know, and I would like to share my own personal life as a demonstration that it has been happening to me. It continues to happen so long as I continue to work on my own personal growth and the expansion of my consciousness through some of the techniques described in this book.

I grew up in a middle-class home in New York, and I was indoctrinated into what has become a very common set of values in society. Those values said that a man must be strong and aggressive; that he must be prepared to be a pillar of the community and the strength of the family; and that he must have a good job, save money, and educate himself to be prepared for work in life. My awareness of others was that we are all different, unique beings, that there is a limited supply of all resources, and that competition determines who gets the biggest pieces of the pie.

The collection of fears, anxieties, tensions, frustrations, anger, hostility, depression, worry, and other emotional responses (so common with most people, though the form may vary for each person) were an everyday part of my life, in spite of my achieving certain accepted worldly signs of success.

So I went about obtaining a strong set of academic credentials in order to prepare myself for the competition, and I received advanced degrees in the social sciences, business sciences, and psychology. At the same time, the training prepared me to think analytically and scientifically, which proved to be of great use in my current career in the healing arts.

In my business career, I rose to the position of executive vice-president of a major cosmetics company. Thus, by all outward signs, I was considered successful.

But my path changed rather abruptly, along with my personal life, when I embarked on my current career in holistic health in another country. However, the same concerns that had dogged me all my life contrived to follow me in whatever I did. All my experience as a psychologist and all the insights gained through psychoanalysis, while helpful, did not relieve the stresses that still followed me.

Changes began about seven years ago when I seemed to have reached my absolute low point. The way of life I thought was real was not providing me with the peace, joy, and love one hears and reads so much about. Not having been religious since the age of thirteen, I rejected the thought of God as a path for me. I wasn't sure I believed in such a Being, anyhow.

Through the suggestion of my brother, who had begun to meditate each day and had found relief from many stressed feelings that had accumulated over the years, I began to meditate as well. This was the start of an extraordinary experience of the transformation of my own consciousness, a transformation that is still occurring.

At first, I attributed the changes to the meditation method itself, but I learned that it was merely a step, a gentle hand that turned the knob of a door that opened for me. As I entered with some caution, new people began to appear in my life; new thoughts and ideas moved in, and I began attending meetings and conferences that brought me further into contact with illuminating ideas and inspiring people.

It was as if the scope of my vision had widened: I was seeing different things than I had seen before about the nature of the world. As part of this continued awareness, I was becoming more willing to listen, to learn, and to deal with the periodic conflicts that would arise between my experiences and the academic training I had received. About five years ago, I met someone who shared with me some spiritual material called *A Course in Miracles.* In an extraordinary experience lasting about ten years this material was received as a kind of "inner dictation" by a highly respected psychologist working in a well-known medical institution. As she describes herself: "Psychologist, educator, conservative in theory and atheistic in belief, I was working in a prestigious and highly academic setting. And then something happened that triggered a chain of events I could never have predicted—the head of my department unexpectedly announced that he was tired of the angry and aggressive feelings our attitudes reflected, and concluded that, 'there must be another way.' As if on cue, I agreed to help him find it. Apparently this *Course* is the other way." The *Course* (1975) is a teaching device consisting of three books: a *Text,* a *Workbook* and a *Manual for Teachers.* The way they are used or studied depends on a persons's needs and preferences.

The curriculum proposed is both theoretical and practical. It specifically states that "a universal theology is impossible, but a universal experience is not only possible but necessary." The *Course* deals with universal spiritual themes. It emphasizes that it is but one form of the universal curriculum. All forms lead to God in the end.

The *Text* is mostly theoretical, providing the concepts on which the course is based. Its ideas form the foundation for the *Workbook's* lessons. The *Workbook* consists of 365 lessons, one for each day of the year. It is practical in emphasizing experience through application as is evident from the introduction to its lessons.

> Some of the ideas the *Workbook* presents you will find hard to believe, and others may seem to be quite startling. This does not matter. You are merely asked to apply the ideas as you are directed to do. You are not asked to judge them at all. You are asked only to use them. It is their use that will give them meaning to you, and will show you that they are true.
>
> Remember only this; you need not believe the ideas, you need not accept them, and you need not even welcome them. Some of them you may actively resist. None of this will matter, or decrease their efficacy. But do not allow yourself to make exceptions in applying the ideas the workbook contains, and whatever your reactions to the ideas may be, use them. Nothing more than that is required.

The *Manual for Teachers* provides answers to some questions a student is likely to ask. It also clarifies some of the terms the *Course* uses.

The *Course* makes no claim to finality or completion of a student's learning. At the end, the student is left in the hands of his or her own Internal Teacher, who directs all further learning as He sees fit.

The *Course* material has changed my life. It has helped me to realize that the world I see is the world I have created through my misperceptions. There is the opportunity to learn and be guided to a more loving, caring, and feeling world where we are all one and are connected with each other as brothers and sisters, stemming from and being of the same Source from which we were all created.

It has given me the realization that we are more than just a body, that we are also a mind and a spirit that is eternal, that we are only limited by those limitations we have imposed on ourselves.

In the symbolic message delivered in my favorite divinely inspired masterpiece, *Jonathan Livingston Seagull* (Bach, 1970), Jonathan says to his fellow gulls:

Each of us is in truth an idea of the Great Gull, an unlimited idea of freedom. . . . Everything that limits us we have to put aside. . . .

Your whole body from wingtip to wingtip . . . is nothing more than your thought itself, in a form you can see. Break the chains of your thought, and you break the chains of your body too. . . ."

Symbolically, *A Course in Miracles* delivers a message I have learned that each of us has an Internal Teacher who is ready to lead us to the right answer at any given moment, if we ask and then listen. The feelings of guilt and sin and other negative thoughts that have, at times, caused me to behave as I do are merely mistakes in perception. They are thoughts that I can correct and change. These misperceptions are barriers to the recognition of Love within me and within all other beings. Recognizing that all-encompassing Love, I can now see my brothers in a totally new light. I now see them as one with me. I try to see that the opposite of Love is fear and that when I see anger, behind it is someone who is scared and is reaching out in the only way he knows how. By constantly reminding myself of this, it has helped me to find the connection between us rather than what appears to separate us.

We are all individual expressions of that unity, and each of us has a part to play in the scenario of life, whether he or she is a truck driver or a college president, a physician or a laborer. Some are further evolved as teachers, here to help those who need to learn. But the teaching is not what we are accustomed to know as teaching. Rather, it is "learning to be what we teach."

Therefore, those who teach are also students, teaching lessons they need to learn. The lesson may not be what is apparent in the form of the material but rather in the substance, the rich source that communicates some universal principle of love, caring, or joining with another in a holy relationship.

In terms of personal change, the message I hear is that we need to stop trying to change the world and one another and to focus on the only true place where anything can change. And that is to *change ourselves*—first. If we are reaching our higher

Source or God, as I understand Him to be, by the personal experience we have with our spiritual Self, then we will be saying and doing whatever is necessary at any given moment to fulfill the Divine Order that is our destiny.

It matters not whether one is Christian, Jew, Moslem, or atheist. All people believe in some force that puts the fragrance in a flower, the life in a seed, the song in a bird, the color in a leaf, and joy and love in the hearts of men. All specialties, all fields of human study, are really facets of the same thing: the human being as part of the universal order of all life. We may seek different paths, but all lead to the same eventual Source.

It is like climbing up a pyramid. There are four sides from which to choose, and there are many paths on each side. Some go more directly to the top; others take a more indirect route. The base is wide, and from it, the view is limited. The other sides cannot be seen. We choose the side and the path we take. As we climb, the sides get more narrow, and the view widens. There is always an option to change paths and accelerate the climb. As we reach for the top, differences narrow, until we begin to see the convergence.

Eventually, we reach the uppermost part, where all sides and all paths join and become one—all sides are visible. It doesn't matter which side or which path we choose, as long as we remember that it is not the side or path that is important but to aim to reach the top.

Mankind may be closer to the top than ever before. Looking down, the fall to the bottom is steeper and more disastrous. But, looking up, the view is unlimited and the splendor supreme.

Each one of us can get glimpses of the beauty near the top in our own lives. It takes daily effort for me to experience those precious moments or "holy instants" of higher consciousness when I listen to my Higher Voice. As I continue to un-learn, by correcting those thoughts that block my awareness of the presence of Love in me, my ego constantly tries to look down instead of up, to see illusions instead of vision.

However, I have found that daily focusing, by meditating, reading the Daily Word, and by doing a prescribed lesson from the *Course,* has provided me with immense rewards in my daily life. There seems to be a cumulative effect, and, although I do slip back into my old consciousness periodically, its impact has weakened and fades quickly.

Find your own path and work on your own consciousness. Therein, you will continue to unfold with the joy, beauty, and love in your life. The future starts now. Letting go of the past releases the present moment where the seeds of the future are sown. The thoughts of today are the events of tomorrow. We create our own reality, and we can be free when we remove the blocks to the awareness of the presence of Love in all of us. That is what we truly are.

Perhaps this book has helped in some way to suggest to you that there is a better way and that the path to finding it is a heightened awareness of yourself in the search for greater meaning in your life. I know that in my life I am an extension of God, at one with all the universe, as we all are. Each of us has a role to perform here on earth and lessons to learn that will help us to grow in increased awareness of who we really are—Children of God.

This holy instant would I give to You.
Be You in charge. For I would follow You,
Certain that Your direction gives me peace.

Lesson 365
A Course in Miracles

Epilogue

ELISABETH KÜBLER-ROSS, M.D.

It is a great pleasure for me to add a few words to those of the outstanding contributors to Elliott Goldwag's book. They have described not only the dilemma of health care but have also shared some optimistic, positive, and hopeful notes about the new direction in which the whole health system is going.

During the past few decades, the science of medicine has made enormous advances. Although many years may not have been added to the life span of man, we have been able to decrease the mortality of children and to prolong man's life with life-sustaining support systems, saving many lives from results of accidents and coronaries. With the help of organ transplants and monitoring devices, we have added to the lives of many who needed more time to finish their "unfinished business" and to pursue their own destinies.

There have been dramatic changes in both the science and the technology of medicine. An enormous amount of knowledge must be accumulated by medical students and physicians to keep up-to-date with all the changes—not only in technology but also in biochemistry and the understanding of disease processes. Probably because of this we have become quite calloused, with less time being spent with the patient as a person.

Very few physicians are able to tell details of a family history or of the standard of living of a given patient—although, they may know the blood count, the size of the liver, and other physical details of their client. This is not a criticism of the physician. It is a factual statement. With the increase of scientific knowledge, the art of medicine has become somewhat lost. I have witnessed this during my practice over the past 20 years Working with dying patients in different university settings across the country, I have been stunned by the inability of many hospital personnel to acknowledge the fact that a patient is beyond medical help. Consequently, they are unable to give assistance to patients and families in making appropriate choices for the final care of loved ones.

When I refer to choices in the final care of loved ones, I mean the options available to patients. Attempts can be made to prolong life within a hospital environment, sustained by life-supporting equipment. Or, one can acknowledge the fact that the science of medicine has done its best; then, the patient could be discharged to spend his last few weeks or days at home with family and friends. It is on very rare occasions that a physician offers these options to a patient and facilitates the transfer of the dying patient to the home. Yet, at home, with the help of visiting nurses, a physician who is willing to make a house call or two, and friends, neighbors, and relatives, the patient's final days can be made as comfortable and as pleasant as possible.

It is mandatory that our patients be cared for so that they are not only pain free but also alert. Since the beginning of the use of the Brompton Mixture (see Appendix B for information), we have been able to take 98 percent of all our terminally ill patients home to die. The oral Brompton Mixture does not contain any heroin, unlike the English version, which does. It has the advantage of keeping our dying patients free of pain and fully conscious until the last few moments of their lives. This makes counseling of emotional and spiritual matters possible. It also enables the dying patient to reevaluate his life, "to finish unfinished business," to communicate with loved ones, and to contribute to his final decision and choices of the final hours and days of his physical existence.

Within this field of caring for the dying patient and his family, there is a tremendous need for more education. Our seminars at the University of Chicago and the ensuing books (Ross 1969, 1974, 1975, 1978) have caused more and more health professionals to become aware of this need. And there has been great change in this field since a decade ago when we were the only group teaching courses on death and dying to medical students and other health professionals. Now, I am delighted to see the new evolving field of thanatology being pursued by so many professionals and laypeople.

During our crusade for this new field of medicine in the last decade, I have traveled about a quarter of a million airline miles annually, reaching approximately 15,000 people a week. We are beginning to see the results of our concerted efforts. There were 120,000 courses on death and dying presented last year in the United States alone. In addition, many lectures have been given by physicians, clergy, psychologists, counselors, nurses, and other health professionals. This has included funeral directors and volunteer organizations such as "The Candlelighters," "The Compassionate Friends," and "Make Today Count." We have covered large geographical areas where the needs of the dying patients are beginning to be met.

About 100 hospices have been established in the United States, some functioning, others in different stages of development. As is always true in any field where the progress and enthusiasm are great, there is the concern that hospices may develop for political and financial benefits. My concern, too, is that many people who have attended our one-week workshops, heard a few lectures, and read my books may begin to claim to be experts and decide to take charge of such facilities.

Yet, they do not have the experience and ability to really carry through with this great responsibility. In order to work in this field, it is of utmost importance to have not only a practical working experience with dying children or adults but also to have an understanding of the important symbolic verbal and non-verbal language that those patients use. The practitioner must be familiar with Susan Bach's *Interpretation of Spontaneous Drawings of Terminally Ill Patients*. He or she must be solidly convinced of the necessity of a total person approach, not only at the end of human life but from the very beginning. We must ensure the quality and dedication of those choosing to enter this new field. Only as we develop in this new field of service with the slow-motion process of evolution, not revolution, are we going to progress in a positive, helpful manner and avoid premature collapse.

Professionals as well as laypeople participate in our one-week live-in workshop retreats given by myself and my staff across the country throughout the year. We are trying to teach all the lessons we have learned from the dying patients and also put the participants personally through a tumbler of experiences to make them aware of their own fears and anxieties as well as unfinished business. Only when our own pool of repressed grief, pain, anxiety, and fear is emptied are we able to work compassionately with patients and their families without becoming exhausted. Otherwise, we carry our unexpressed feelings from the sick room and externalize them to undeserving people, such as staff or family members. A form of psychodrama used in our one-week workshops facilitates the upsurge of negative feelings, which can then be expressed and shared with the group. In return, the listeners can get in touch with their own unfinished business.

Our workshops are attended by many seeking help—such as the 14-year-old suicidal child as well as the 93-year-old lady who is trying to come to grips with her own impending death. Dying patients, many multiple sclerosis patients, and quadraplegics participate in these workshops. So do the parents of dying, murdered, or suicidal children. The professional and the patient are brought together to share their points of view, their philosophies, and their problems. As they begin to recognize mutual concerns and difficulties, they become aware that we are all human beings with a facet of divinity within. They begin to see that we each have all the assets to choose our destinies and to become whole.

In this new era of holistic medicine, we are finally beginning to appreciate that the human being is not only a physical body but consists of an intellectual, emotional, physical, and spiritual quadrant. It is only as we come into harmony within these four quadrants and accept our *natural* emotions that we become truly whole and healthy. The physician of the next decade will learn more about the emotional and spiritual quadrants and how he can facilitate this harmony by getting involved with the total person. It is hoped that more physicians, nurses, therapists, social workers, and other health professionals will reevaluate their practices and their understanding of the person. Expectantly, their comprehension of what health really means will be better defined and broadened, and they will begin to take time to listen to the human being in order to understand where his ill health is coming from.

It is far easier, quicker, and more economically feasible to sedate parents in an emergency room when they have been told of the accidental death of their young child. A prescription of Valium takes two minutes, and the family can be sent home after they have signed the consent papers. What we do not seem to comprehend fully in this type of situation, however, is that we are always totally responsible for the consequences of our choices. We are responsible for the grief and pain and unexpressed anguish that many of these parents carry with them for months and even years until they need expensive, time-consuming psychiatric help. The obvious alternative is to allow family members of sudden-death victims to express their pain immediately after being informed of the tragedy. They need not be sedated! Instead, they should be taken to a separate, private room adjacent to the emergency room, which we call the "screaming" room. There, the help of a compassionate friend who, it is hoped, has come through a similar life experience can facilitate the externalization of the family's pain and be available for questions without the family having to be sedated. The family should also be encouraged to view the body after it has been cleaned and bandaged but still recognizable. The grief process can be greatly shortened by following this procedure. Most of these families will never require psychiatric help or show prolonged and pathological grief after the loss of a loved one.

The necessity of screaming rooms has been verified during the 12 years of our work with families of sudden-death victims. They have also proved equally important for the hospital staff in ventilating some of the negative feelings that come up in a very demanding job where there is very little time for expression of one's own anguish. Nurses, chaplains, physicians, and social workers should have access to and make use of the screaming room as well when their "buckets are full." If they have an understanding and nonjudgmental partner in the room with them, they can externalize their frustration. To get rid of normal, natural anger or frustration does not take more than 15 seconds. Then, they can resume their work with a cheerful disposition and leave at the end of the day without feeling drained and exhausted. From a purely economical point of view, this procedure has proved to be very valuable within the administration of the hospital, too. Sick leaves have become less frequent. The turnover of nursing staff, especially in intensive care units, has also diminished rapidly. These types of changes within health care not only help bereaved families and those who are dying but also make the work for the hospital personnel more enjoyable and less draining.

At Shanti Nilaya, our new growth and healing center in Escondido, California, we have established a place of retreat for all those who need to "recharge their batteries." Opportunities are presented for the participants to take a look at their motivations and wants and to begin to live fully without fear of their own or their loved ones' death. We feel the work at this center is vitally important for health professionals as well as their terminally ill patients and their families. We encourage all to visit the center and attend our one-week retreat workshops. Within the next decade, we plan to have such a center in every state so that these services will be available to more and more people, without the need for long-distance traveling.

Elliott Goldwag's book is a beautiful summary by health professionals who have had the courage to stick out their necks. They have studied the whole person and each, in his own way, has contributed to a better understanding of man and man's health as can be seen from the total person view.

I congratulate all the contributors of this book but especially Elliott Goldwag. Our hope is that many health professionals and laypeople will read this book and become encouraged to have faith about the direction health care is taking and venture forth to become leaders in this new era of holistic health. We are hopeful of a future no longer dominated by economic disasters and sedating drugs for the terminally ill but by reasonable and economical care of the *total* person, with a peaceful acceptance of the coming of death—a simple transition into another form of life.

A City of Health: Model of a Holistic Health Center

ELLIOTT M. GOLDWAG, Ph.D.

The growing awareness that health is the result of the body, mind, and spirit in harmony and balance is encouraging the emergence of new forms of health care centers. These centers differ considerably from the more traditional crisis-care or disease-care centers to which we in the United States have grown accustomed in the past few years.

A number of hybrid organizations have appeared, calling themselves "holistic health" or "wellness" centers. These centers have been interpreted by some to mean a group of practitioners gathered together in a common building or located within close proximity of one another to serve as a cross-referral group for people needing various types of therapy.

Other centers have developed to revolve around one key professional whose primary interest may be in nutrition, exercise, psychotherapy, or body therapies—that is, bioenergetics, gestalt therapy, and so on. Here, the emphasis is on the mode of

322

treatment within the particular orientation of the therapist, although other therapies may also be utilized.

PHILOSOPHY OF CITY OF HEALTH

Although called a "city," this health care model does not necessarily include a community wherein people reside but refers rather to a diversified center wherein many types of activities can be offered.

This idea for such a center began germinating in my mind a number of years ago, influenced greatly by my experiences with the Renaissance Revitalization Center in Nassau, Bahamas. This health-oriented center was co-founded by my brother, Dr. William Goldwag; Dr. Ivan Popov, a physician from Europe; and myself.

Many of the ideas presented here were originally intended to be developed for a center to be located in Houston, Texas, where many professionals, interested nonprofessionals, and spiritual leaders believed the first working model could and should be. As of this date, such a project has not come to fruition there, although the principles outlined here are applicable to any other part of the country as well as to Houston.

The formation of such a center is deeply rooted in many of the ideas expressed throughout this book:

1. A human being is a whole person, more than the sum of his parts.
2. Good health results from the inner balance of the body, mind, and spirit of each person.
3. The enemy of good health is stress. Stress is the response a person chooses as a reaction to a given situation. Everyone responds differently, depending upon the perception of the world he or she chooses to see. Since perception is the result of an individual's belief system, it is in this area that the initial cause of illness and disease is to be found.
4. Toxic germs, or toxic ideas, lead to stress and cause biochemical, physiological, and psychological changes in the body. Such changes attack the immune system, lower the level of resistance, and enable viruses and bacteria to begin the disease process.

5. Two major services are necessary for the person who is ill:

Relief of the symptoms.

Help to prevent futher recurrence of the illness.

6. Everyone is a participant in his or her illness process; therefore, we each should be a participant in the process of getting well and staying that way.

7. All treatments are temporary expedients until a person is helped to understand how his or her thoughts and belief systems influence his or her health. Faith, no matter what its form, is the basis of individual spiritual expression which each of us has. It is the Faith, Hope, and Love that Marcus Bach describes which forms the cornerstone of a holistic center (see Chapter 9).

8. Through a holistic philosophy, guidance can be given to help people help themselves.

FUNCTION OF CITY OF HEALTH

There are three main aspects of the center's function. Thanks go to my friends, Dr. Grant Taylor and Dr. Fred Elliott of Houston, for suggesting how these functions may be represented in diagrammatic form:

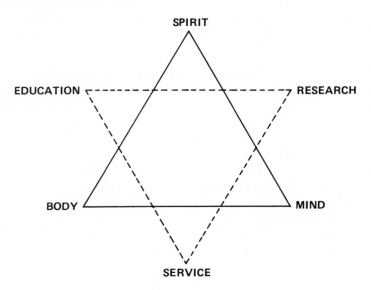

This star formation highlights the wholeness of man—spirit, body, and mind—and the three facets of the City of Health— service, education, and research.

Service

The pivotal point of service is twofold—the staff to provide help and the kind of help to be offered. The key to the success of any health-oriented center is a careful selection of proper personnel. The staff is far more than a collection of persons with professional skills, however. Each member is actively participating in his own "wholeness," or higher consciousness, achieving his own *inner balance.*

There are no hierarchical divisions deifying one profession over another. The teamwork approach is visualized within the City of Health where loving, caring people form a treatment group. Since the primary person normally responsible for health care in the United States is the physician, this individual forms the nucleus of the treatment group. Within this framework, the art of medicine is ensured an equal role with the science of medicine. An interdisciplinary approach is encouraged in order to use the valuable contributions of nurses, social workers, psychotherapists, pastoral counselors, and other professionals and paraprofessionals. The major objective is always: *Help people help themselves.*

The City of Health staff also recognizes that no one therapist or single therapy is necessarily the catalyst for healing but rather that a multitherapeutic approach is the most effective program. With this understanding, the staff works in harmony with one another without the interference of personal ego clouding the attitude of wholeness that prevails.

Traditional and nontraditional approaches to healing are incorporated in a responsible manner, under responsible supervision. With prevention as the primary goal, encouragement of personal responsibility and growth is the keystone to such an objective. Clients are able to broaden their awareness of how self-direction and self-realization can enrich their lives and change a debilitating lifestyle to one of health and substance.

Those participating in the various programs of the City of Health are helped to understand how to initiate personal change and how to sustain such change. Methods of coping with life-style pressures and how one can see them differently are incorporated. An opportunity for self-realization and discovery is essential in the center's treatment program. A variety of modalities are used to implement this process, including such services as biofeedback, educational classes, meditation training, various psychotherapeutic experiences, yoga, spiritual counseling, and nutrition evaluation and training, to name a few. Services, of course, provide traditional medical evaluation and appraisal as the first step in determining the appropriate program for an individual. The list of services at the center is limited only by its proven worth and appropriateness to the primary goal of health.

Central to all services is the time taken by an understanding staff to listen to the client. The neglect of this important need continues to be the chief complaint patients express about their present medical care whenever surveys are taken of patient attitudes.

The City of Health is not intended to provide acute care services. These are far better supplied by a community hospital or medical center that has the staff and facilities to render such intervention. The vast majority of illnesses or diseases, however, are of a chronic nature, requiring a different kind of regimen to aid in the person's recovery.

Education

Training and education is an exciting component of the City of Health. Such activity provides further growth for the following groups:

The Staff. In order to maintain the goal of wholeness, the staff recognizes and participates in activities promoting their own personal growth. In this way, they heighten their abilities to help themselves and thereby are of greater service to clients.

Clients of the Center. Clients attend classes, view videotapes, use audiovisual aids, borrow books, read pamphlets, and find a ready source of training themselves in better ways of achieving and maintaining their own health and that of their families.

Professionals and Students in the Health Sciences. Opportunities are provided for practicing health professionals to work in residence at the center. By learning how to apply holistic concepts in their own lives and professions, these practitioners can then share these ideas within their own communities for implementation in local health care facilities. Liaisons with medical and other professional schools provide unique opportunities for students to become aware of this type of health care center and of how it functions. Internships are offered in order to assure continuing education of professionals concentrating on health instead of disease.

A continuous flow of information is available to the public concerning the center and its work. Educational materials, along with the published results of research, are provided so that organizations and other interested parties can become aware and remain current with the work at the center.

Research

As ideas evolve in any field, they are refined through testing and evaluation, applying scientific methods for such appraisal. The many new modes of treatment that are proliferating do require careful appraisal regarding their usefulness or validity in any health maintenance program.

The City of Health model incorporates the services of skilled researchers who help to provide these investigative procedures and to facilitate removal of the obscurity surrounding such methods. It is more than likely that the newer forms of treatment or diagnosis that are developed require newer methods of research technology. In some instances, a change in the paradigms we now accept as the scientific method may be necessary. An appreciation of Albert Einstein's statement that one can never remove the observer from the observation prescribes that such researchers be open to new thought and expansion of the horizons of traditional health care.

Constant liaisons with medical institutions in the research effort offer additional dimensions to the center's capabilities to offer service.

With the triangle of service, education, and research (service being the primary function), the City of Health attracts an outstanding staff capable of rendering quality care. It is an important step in achieving balance between crisis intervention and medical repair and in gaining a focus on health and wholeness.

PHYSICAL LOCATION

Ideally, such a center is best located in an esthetic, natural surrounding, removed from the pressure and tension of urban activity. However, there is convenient accessibility to existing crisis-care medical institutions to maintain necessary liaisons. The center is also within easy reach of individuals who are using the services on an out-client basis.

An architectural design reinforcing a natural, relaxed atmosphere of caring is desirable. Effects of natural lighting and a warm decor with furnishings lending themselves to a personal rather than the traditional institutional interior enhances the freedom to become healthy.

Adequate space is provided for various types of therapies—once again, with a decor that is warm, comfortable, and reassuring. A sanctuary for meditation and prayer is a central part of the physical structure. A distinction is made here between spiritual attunement and a particular religious persuasion. Everyone is encouraged to seek his or her own spiritual guidance in whatever path he or she finds most comfortable for his or her own unfoldment.

Sports facilities are also appropriately located on the premises, implementing physical fitness programs considered helpful in health maintenance. Depending upon the physical location of a center, such facilities might include sports activities for individuals and families not otherwise needing the center's other services.

A fine restaurant facility offering gourmet foods, nutritionally planned and prepared, attracts many to the facility. Such a restaurant offers a practical demonstration that food can be nutritionally sound and still delightfully appetizing.

BOARD OF ADVISORS

Centers such as the City of Health are much different from present health care facilities. New ideas are sometimes threatening to existing systems and to people with vested interests in illness models. It is essential to maintain professional integrity and a relationship with traditional medical institutions. The objective should always be to find the common denominators that join people rather than the differences that separate them.

Therefore, it is most desirable to establish a prestigious board of advisors of professionals, spiritual leaders, and laypeople who lend their names and support to the center. This assures the credibility and authenticity of the center's activities. This type of master mind alliance also provides continuous input of new ideas and thoughts from leaders who are in constant touch with what is happening.

SUMMARY

The disease-oriented model that has dominated our high cost national health care system has outlived its usefulness. It needs to be modified. The emerging wave of thought about holistic health reminds us of this need. The "whole" person is a physical, mental, and spiritual being; and unless that person is functioning in balance and harmony, the frequent end product is illness. The consciousness of holistic health promises to be the area where the greatest advances in total health care will be seen. The City of Health is viewed as a facility that focuses attention on new technologies, responsibly researched and developed, and sees that they are made available to consumers and professionals in health care.

A City of Health is the important next step in providing a working success model that demonstrates the feasibility and effectiveness of the ideas discussed here. I believe that other such centers will begin to develop and be established throughout the United States once a model begins to operate. It will probably require private funds to launch the initial City of Health. Once several such locations have proved that there is a need and have become effective, government at both the federal and state levels will then feel secure and will be encouraged to lend its support.

Centers will vary in the form they assume, of course, depending on the location and on the perceived needs of the area. The common denominator in achieving success is always to strive toward the recognition of the need for a greater spiritual awareness among all people. Such growth is the central core in the maintenance of individual health and happiness.

B

Brompton's Mixture For Relief of Pain In Terminal Disease*

K. GREGORY HUMMA, M.S.
WILLIAM M. DUGAN, M.D.
DONNA J. MINNICK

A recent marked increase in the use of the time-honored Brompton's Mixture at the Royal Victoria Hospital in Montreal, Canada, in the relief of terminal cancer pain has led to the need for clarification with respect to what concentrations are available and how to order the appropriate elixir.**

The following points have been established to facilitate achieving optimal control of pain and maximum ease of prescription.

1. All written orders must specify the exact dose of morphine and the name of the phenothiazine required, complying with the standard mixtures available in the hospital pharmacy. Orders such as "Brompton's Mixture" cannot be filled.

---

*Extracted from *A Primer on Brompton's Cocktail*, published by Methodist Hospital, Indianapolis, Indiana. Reprinted by permission.
**See The Canadian Medical Association Journal, Issue of July 17, 1976, Volume No. 115, No. 2.

2. The pharmacy will make available the following standard elixir:

   morphine 10 mg

   cocaine 10 mg

   Ethyl Alcohol 5 cc

   Syrup 5 cc

   Chloroform water ad 20 cc

   Alternative available standard elixirs will contain: morphine 20 mg, morphine 30 mg, or morphine 40 mg, respectively.

3. The standard elixir is always given with a *phenothiazine syrup, which will be added by the medication nurse on the ward.* Prochlorperazine (Stemetil 5 mg in 5 ml) is the one normally added. Chlorpromazine (Largactil 25 mg in 5 ml) may be used if sedation is required. These potentiate the effect of morphine and also act as antiemetics and tranquilizers.

4. 20 cc of the standard elixir plus phenothiazine should be given Q4H around the clock and not prn. The aim is not to relieve pain but to prevent pain and erase the memory of pain by titrating the elixir to the patient's needs, providing coverage regularly at that level. No repeat prescription is permitted for narcotics, and doctors are reminded that their BNDD number must be included on every outside prescription. If the prescription is to be filled at an outside pharmacy, the complete formulas must be written along with instructions. A separate prescription for phenothiazine enables the physician to adjust the dose of this drug to suit the patient's needs. The starting dose would be 5 mg Stemetil or 10 mg of Largactil.

For further information on the use of the Brompton's Mixture, you may contact:

Gregg Humma, M.S.   317–924–8471 or 316–924–8436
Clinical Pharmacist
Department of Pharmacy
Methodist Hospital
1604 North Capitol
Indianapolis, Indiana   46202

The procedures outlined for handling Brompton's Cocktail conform to all Indiana state and federal controlled substance laws and regulations. However, controlled substance laws may vary in different states and these differences should be taken into account when prescribing and dispensing the Brompton's Cocktail.

The three medical oncologists involved in the Brompton's study have submitted a physician-sponsored IND to the Food and Drug Administration.

Since the spring of 1975, more than 150 patients with terminal cancer and chronic pain have been treated with Brompton's Cocktail at Methodist Hospital of Indiana, Inc. As of the present, no double blind controlled studies which delineate the usefulness of Brompton's Cocktail as compared to other analgesic drugs have been published in the literature. The successful use of this drug combination in many patients has prompted Methodist personnel to initiate the planning for such a study.

"A Primer on Brompton's Cocktail" represents a compilation of information gathered in an 18-month period by personnel involved in direct patient care.

Our efforts at Methodist Hospital to use Brompton's Cocktail have been stimulated by Dr. Elisabeth Kübler-Ross, noted physician, psychiatrist, and thanatology expert. To quote Dr. Ross: "There are still thousands of patients who wait much too long for the next injection for pain relief and who are unable to live until they die because their only preoccupation is to get some adequate relief from their suffering."

This information is prepared for medical and allied health personnel with the hope that the suffering of terminally ill patients can be relieved.

Brompton's Cocktail is an oral, liquid analgesic mixture that has been in use in Great Britain and Canada for a number of years. It is listed as an official preparation (Diamorphine and Cocaine Elixir) in both the British Pharmaceutical Codex (1973) and the British National Formulary (1974–76). The British use heroin (diamorphine or diacetylmorphine) in their preparation since it is permissible to use this drug in the treatment of terminal cancer patients in Great Britain.

Experience with Brompton's Cocktail at Methodist dates to early 1975 when one of our nurses returned from an oncology seminar with information on this preparation. Several references to the use of Brompton's Cocktail were located in the literature and Methodist's oncologists became interested in assessing its effectiveness with several of their patients. Initially, Brompton's Cocktail was prepared according to the British formula with the substitution of morphine for heroin and contained in each 20 ml dose:

morphine	10 mg
cocaine	10 mg
ethyl alcohol 95%	5 ml
cherry syrup	5 ml
chloroform water QS	20 ml

Each 20 ml dose was given with a 5 ml dose of Compazine syrup (prochlorperizine) 5 mg/5ml every four hours around the clock on a scheduled basis. It appeared from the literature that Brompton's Cocktail might be more effective in the treatment of pain because of interactions between its various ingredients:

narcotics + alcohol = potentiation
narcotics + phenothiazines = potentiation
alcohol + phenothiazines = potentiation

It was noted quite soon after the use of Brompton's Cocktail was initiated that many patients complained about the taste. The vehicle was changed to Aromatic Elixir (a commercially available preparation of orange oil, lemon oil, coriander oil, anise oil, simple syrup and 22% alcohol) with each 20 ml dose containing the following:

morphine	10 mg
cocaine	10 mg
Aromatic Elixir QS	20 ml

Patient acceptance of this current preparation is much improved.

The strength of morphine in each 20 ml dose of Brompton's Cocktail can be varied by the physician as needed. Some patients on Brompton's Cocktail for extended periods of time have required 40 mg or more of morphine per dose to obtain adequate pain relief. Most patients seem to do well on 10 mg or 20 mg of morphine per dose. Currently none of the physicians at Methodist regularly prescribe the concurrent use of Compazine syrup with Brompton's Cocktail even though nausea remains a problem.

More than 150 terminal cancer patients with chronic pain have been treated at Methodist Hospital with Brompton's Cocktail. At present, a multidisciplinary committee of nurses, physicians, pharmacists and the Associate Program Director of the Clinical Oncology Program has been formed to design and conduct a controlled study to assess the benefits of Brompton's Cocktail in terminal patients. In general, the physicians who have used Brompton's Cocktail in our institution feel that it is very useful in selected patients. The most common side effect seen in patients appears to be drowsiness. This is more pronounced in older patients but generally subsides in a few days. Others include diaphoresis, nausea, vomiting, disorientation, and constipation. Basically the above side effects are common to all narcotics. The particular advantage with the Brompton's Cocktail is that by carefully monitoring individual patient response alterations in the cocktail can provide a pain-free state without sedation. The cocktail is given as often as every three hours or as infrequently as every six (most patients require an every four hour administration). During period of dosage adjustment, supplemental analgesics and antiemetics are used as needed (either parenterally or orally).

Sources of Supply for Various Ingredients in Brompton's Cocktail
A. Morphine
   Morphine sulfate hypodermic tabs – 30 mg

   Eli Lilly & Co.
   Indianapolis, IN
B. Cocaine
   Cocaine hydrochloride crystals
   Cocaine hydrochloride solvets – 160 mg
   Mallinckrodt Pharmaceuticals (crystals)
   St. Louis, Missouri

   Eli Lilly & Co. (solvets)
   Indianapolis, IN
C. Aromatic Elixir
   Eli Lilly & Co. (pints)
   Indianapolis, IN

   Century Pharmaceuticals (gallons)
   Indianapolis, IN

What is Brompton's Cocktail? Brompton's Cocktail is a potent oral analgesic mixture which is used to relieve and prevent the pain associated with selected cases of terminal cancer. The Brompton's Cocktail in use at Methodist is a modification of a formula first used with great success in the cancer hospitals of Great Britain.

What does Brompton's Cocktail consist of and how is it administered? The basic formula for a 20 ml dose of Brompton's Cocktail consists of the following:

morphine	10 mg
cocaine	10 mg
Aromatic Elixir qs ad	20 ml

Aromatic Elixir is a flavoring vehicle consisting of orange oil, lemon oil, anise oil, coriander oil, sugar and about 22% alcohol. The overall flavor is a somewhat sweet orange. The concentration of morphine in each dose may be increased or decreased at the discretion of the physician. Each dose may also be given with a dose of Compazine syrup 5 mg/5 ml. Brompton's Cocktail is administered orally on a scheduled basis usually every four hours around the clock, although this time interval may be varied by the physician.

How does Brompton's Cocktail work in the treatment of pain? In addition to the individual potency of each of the ingredients contained in Brompton's Cocktail, it may be more effective as a combination because each of the active ingredients interacts with others to potentiate the analgesic and CNS depressant actions:

$$\text{narcotics} + \text{alcohol} = \text{potentiation}$$
$$\text{narcotics} + \text{phenothiazines} = \text{potentiation}$$
$$\text{phenothiazines} + \text{alcohol} = \text{potentiation}$$

Some patients taking Brompton's Cocktail may still require narcotic injections as a "back-up" or for the first few days of treatment until a high enough narcotic blood level is obtained.

What are some of the Side effects that may occur with Brompton's Cocktail? The major side effects that might be seen with Brompton's Cocktail include respiratory depression, constipation, and drowsiness. Some patients have complained of a burning sensation when swallowing Brompton's Cocktail, which is probably due to the relatively high alcohol content.

Bibliography

Chapter 1

Beecher, H. K. Evidence for Increased Effectiveness of Placebos With Increased Stress. *American Journal of Physiology,* 1956, 187, 163–169.

Bernard, C. *An Introduction to the Study of Experimental Medicine.* New York: Macmillan, 1927.

Boudreau, T. A New Perspective on the Health of Canadians. *Conference on Future Directions in Health Care.* December 10–11, 1975. Waldorf Astoria, New York, N.Y.

Cannon, W. B. *The Wisdom of the Body.* New York: W. W. Norton & Co., 1939.

Carrel, A. *Man The Unknown.* New York: Harper & Bros., 1935.

Dubos, R. *The Mirage of Health.* New York: Harper & Bros., 1959.

Engel, G. L. *Psychological Development in Health and Disease.* Philadelphia: W. B. Saunders Co., 1962.

Frank, J. D. *Persuasion and Healing.* Baltimore: Johns Hopkins University Press, 1973.

337

Freud, S. *A General Introduction to Psychoanalysis.* Garden City, New York: Garden City Publishing Co., 1943.

Haas, Fink & Hartfelder. *Pharmacology Service Center Bulletin,* Vol. 2, July 1963.

Halstead, L. S. & Halstead, M. G. Chronic Illness and Humanism: Rehabilitation as a Model for Teaching Humanistic Health Care. *Archives of Physical Medicine and Rehabilitation,* 1978, 59, 53-57.

Moser, R. *Internal Medicine Reporter,* Stanford, Conn.: Jan. 1976.

Palmer, R. E. The AMA's Health Plan. *Newsweek,* Jan. 6, 1977, p. 11.

Thomas, L. *The Lives of a Cell.* New York: The Viking Press, 1974.

Tinbergen, N. Ethology and Stress Diseases. *Science,* 1974, 185.

Vallery-Radot, M. R. *The Life of Pasteur* (R. L. Devonshire, trans. with an introd. by Sir William Osler). Garden City, N.Y.: Garden City Publishing Co., 1923.

Virchow, R. *Disease, Life and Man.* (L. J. Rather, Ed. and trans.). Stanford, California: Stanford University Press, 1958, 18.

Wolf, S. *Behavioral Science in Clinical Medicine.* Springfield, Illinois: Charles C. Thomas, 1976.

Chapter 2

Albrecht, K. *Stress and the Manager.* Englewood Cliffs, New Jersey: Prentice-Hall, in press.

Blythe, P. *Stress Disease, The Growing Plague.* New York: St. Martin's Press, 1973.

Cannon, W. B. *The Wisdom of the Body.* New York: W. W. Norton & Co., 1939.

Friedman, M. & Rosenman, R. H. *Type A Behavior and Your Heart.* New York: Alfred A. Knopf, 1974.

Knowles, J. H. (Ed.). *Doing Better and Feeling Worse.* New York: W. W. Norton & Co., 1977.

Lamott, K. *Escape From Stress. How to Stop Killing Yourself.* New York: G. P. Putnam's Sons, 1974.

Levi, L. & Andersson, L. Population, Environment and Quality of Life. *Ekistics,* July, 1975, 236, 12-19.

McQuade, W. & Aikman, A. *Stress, What It Is, What It Can Do To Your Health, How To Fight Back.* New York: E. P. Dutton & Company, Inc., 1974.

Sarason, I. G. & Spielberger, C.D. (Eds.). *Stress and Anxiety* (Vol. 3). Washington-London: Hemisphere Publishing Corp., 1976.

Selye, H. *Experimental Cardiovascular Diseases.* Berlin-Heidelberg-New York: Springer-Verlag, 1970.

Selye, H. *Hormones & Resistance.* Berlin-Heidelberg-New York: Springer-Verlag, 1971.

Selye, H. *Stress in Health and Disease.* Reading, Massachusetts: Butterworths, 1976.

Selye, H. *Stress Without Distress.* Philadelphia: J. B. Lippincott Co., 1974.

Selye, H. *The Stress of Life* (1st ed.). New York: McGraw-Hill Book Co., 1956. 2nd ed., 1976.

Tanner, O. *Human Behavior: Stress.* New York: Time-Life Books, 1976.

Wolf, S. & Goodell, H. *Behavioral Science in Clinical Medicine.* Springfield, Illinois: Charles C. Thomas, 1976.

Wolf, S. & Goodell, H. *Stress and Disease* (2nd ed.). Springfield, Illinois: Charles C. Thomas, 1968.

Chapter 3

Albrecht, K. *Stress and the Manager.* Englewood Cliffs, New Jersey: Prentice Hall, 1979.

Basowitz, H., Persky, H., Korchin, S. J. & Grinker, R. R. *Anxiety and Stress.* New York: McGraw-Hill Book Co., 1955.

Braunwald, E. Future Shock in Academic Medicine. New England Journal of Medicine, 1972, 286, 1031-1035.

Brown, B. B. *Stress and the Art of Biofeedback.* New York: Harper & Row, 1977.

Cannon, W. B. *The Wisdom of the Body.* New York: W. W. Norton & Co., 1939.

Engel, G. L. The Need For a New Medical Model: A Challenge for Biomedicine. *Science,* 1977, 196, 129-136.

Luthe, W. *Stress and Self-Regulation: Introduction to the Methods of Autogenic Therapy.* Montreal: Workshop Manual of the International Institute of Stress, 1977.

McQuade, W. & Aikman, A. *Stress. What It Is. What It Can Do To Your Health. How To Fight Back.* New York: E. P. Dutton & Co., 1974.

Oates, Jr., R. M. (Ed.). *Celebrating the Dawn. Maharishi Mahesh Yogi and the TM Technique.* New York: G. Putnam's Sons, 1976.

Roskies, E. & Lazarus, R. S. Coping Theory and the Teaching of Coping Skills. In P. Davidson, Ed., *Behavioral Medicine: Changing Health Life Styles.* New York: Brunner/Mazel, in press.

Rossier, J., Bloom, F. E. & Guillemin, R. Endorphins and Stress. In H. Selye, *Guide to Stress Research.* New York: Van Nostrand Reinhold, in press.

Schuller, R. H. *Turning Your Stress Into Strength.* Irvine, California: Harvest House, 1978.

Selye, H. *From Dream to Discovery.* New York: Arno Press, 1975.

Selye, H. *Stress in Health and Disease.* Reading, Massachusetts: Butterworths, 1976.

Selye, H. *Stress Without Distress.* Philadelphia: J. B. Lippincott Co., 1974.

Selye, H. *The Stress of Life* (1st ed.). New York: McGraw-Hill Book Co., 1956, (2nd ed.) 1976.

Selye, H. *The Stress of MY Life.* Toronto: McClelland & Stewart, 1977.

Truch, S. *The TM Technique and the Art of Learning.* Toronto: Lester & Orpen Ltd., 1977.

Wolff, H. G. *The Mind-Body Relationship. An Outline of Man's Knowledge.* New York: Doubleday, 1960.

Wolf, S. & Goodell. S. *Behavioral Science in Clinical Medicine.* Springfield, Illinois: Charles C. Thomas, 1976.

Wolf, S. & Goodell, S. *Behavioral Science in Clinical Medicine.* Springfield, Charles C. Thomas, 1968.

Chapter 4

Benson, H. *The Relaxation Response.* New York: William Morrow, 1973.

Biofeedback Society of America Task Force Reports, 1977. (Available from: Biofeedback Society of America, Francine Butler, Executive Secretary, Univ. of Colorado Medical Center, 4200 East 9th Ave., Denver, CO 80220)

Brown, B. Recognition of aspects of consciousness through association with EEG alpha activity represented by a light signal. *Psychophysiology,* 6:442, 1970.

Carrington, P. *Clinically Standardized Meditation.* Kendall Park, N.J.: Pace Books, 1978.

Carrington, P. *Freedom in Meditation.* New York: Anchor Press, 1977.

Fehmi, L. G. Open Focus Training. A paper presented in a workshop at Council Grove Conference on Voluntary Control of Internal States, April 3, 1975, Council Grove, Kansas. Paper available from author, 905 Herrontown Road, Princeton, N.J. 08540.

Glueck, B. C. Biofeedback and Meditation in the Treatment of Psychiatric Illnesses. *Comprehensive Psychiatry*, 1975, 16.

Green, E. & Green, A. *Beyond Biofeedback.* New York: Delacorte, 1977.

Jacobson, E. *You Must Relax.* New York: McGraw Hill, 1978.

James, W. *The Letters of William James* (Vol. 2). H. James, Ed. Boston: Atlantic Monthly Press, 1920, pp. 253-254. (Reprinted in *William James on Psychical Research,* Murphy & Ballou (Eds.). New York: Viking Press, 1960.

Kamiya, J. Operant Control of EEG Alpha Rhythm and Some of Its Reported Effects on Consciousness. In C. T. Tart (Ed.), *Altered States of Consciousness.* New York: John Wiley & Sons, 1969.

Lamott, K. *Escape From Stress.* New York: G. P. Putnam, 1975.

Menninger, K. Healthier than Healthy. In E. B. Hall (Ed.), *A Psychiatrist's World: The Selected Papers of Karl Menninger, M.D.* New York: The Viking Press, 1959.

Miller, N. Learning of visceral and glandular responses. *Science,* 163:434, 1969.

Pelletier, K. R. *Mind As Healer, Mind As Slayer.* New York: Delta, 1977.

Schultz, J. H. & Luthe, W. *Autogenic Training.* New York: Grune & Stratton, 1959.

Selye, H. *Stress Without Distress.* Philadelphia: Lippincott, 1974.

Stress and Behavioral Medicine (Vol. 1 & 2). New York: Biomonitoring Applications Publications, 1977-1978.

Stroebel, C. F. Biofeedback Procedures. In *Biofeedback and Behavioral Medicine: Current Applications and Prospects.* New York: Biomonitoring Applications Publications, 1978.

Stroebel, C. F. *Clinical Biofeedback and Vasoconstrictive Syndromes.* New York: Biomonitoring Applications Publications, 1976.

Stroebel, C. F. Placebo Effects in Biofeedback Training. In *Biofeedback Techniques in Clinical Practice.* New York: Biomonitoring Applications Publications, 1977.

Stroebel, C. F. *The Quieting Response.* New York: Biomonitoring Applications Publications, 1978.

Stroebel, C. F. & Glueck, B. C. Biofeedback Treatment in Medicine and Psychiatry: An Ultimate Placebo? *Seminars in Psychiatry*, Vol. 5, 1973.

Stroebel, C. F. & Glueck, B. C. Passive Meditation: Subjective Clinical and Electrographic Comparison with Biofeedback. In G. E. Schwartz & D. Shapiro (Eds.), *Consciousness and Self Regulation* (Vol. 2). New York: Plenum Publishing Corp., 1978.

Stroebel, C. F. & Glueck, B. C. Psychophysiological Rationale for the Application of Biofeedback in the Alleviation of Pain. In *Pain: New Perspectives in Therapy and Research*. New York: Plenum, 1976.

Stroebel, C. F., Glueck, B. C., McKnight, R., et al. *Biofeedback Protocol*. Hartford, Connecticut: Institute of Living, 1977.

Stroebel, C. F., Luce, G. G. & Glueck, B. C. *Psychophysiological Diary: A Computer Scored Daily Record of Moods, Body Changes and Life Events*. Hartford, Conn.: Institute of Living, 1971.

Tzu, Lao. *The Way of Life* (W. Bynner, trans.). New York: Capricorn Books, 1944.

Whatmore, G. & Kohli, D. *The Physiology and Treatment of Functional Disorders*. New York: Grune & Stratton, 1974.

Chapter 5

Abdullah, S. & Schucman, H. Cerebral Lateralization, Bimodal Consciousness & Related Developments in Psychiatry. *Research Communications in Psychology, Psychiatry and Behavior*. 1976, Vol., 1 #5 and 6, 671–679.

Benson, H. *Relaxation Response*. New York: William Morrow, 1975.

Benson, H. & Wallace, K. R. Decreased drug abuse with transcendental meditation: a study of 1,862 subjects, in Drug Abuse. *Proceedings of the International Conference*. C. Zarafonetis (Ed.). Philadelphia: Lea and Febiger, 1972, 369–376.

Deikman, A. J. Bimodal Consciousness. *Archives General Psychiatry*, Vol. 25, Dec. 1971.

Editorial. Meditation of Methyldopa? *British Medical Journal*. London: June, 1976.

Galin, D. Implications for Psychiatry of Left and Right Cerebral Specialization. *Archives General Psychiatry*, Vol. 31, Oct. 1974.

Galin, D. & Ornstein, R. Lateral Specialization of Cognitive Mode: An EEG Study. *Psychophysiology*, Vol. 9, #4, 1972.

Gersten, D. J. Meditation as an Adjunct to Medical and Psychiatric Treatment. *American Journal of Psychiatry,* Vol. 135, 5, May, 1978.

Glueck, B. C. & Stroebel, C. F. Biofeedback and Meditation in the Treatment of Psychiatric Illnesses. *Comprehensive Psychiatry,* July-Aug. 1975, Vol. 16 (4); 304–321.

Green, E. E., Green, A. M., & Walters, E. D. Voluntary Control of Inner States: Psychological and Physiological. *Journal of Transpersonal Psychology.* 1970, Vol. 2 (1).

Jacobson, E. *Anxiety and Tension Control.* Philadelphia: J. P. Lippincott, 1964.

LeShan, L. *The Medium, the Mystic, and the Physicist.* New York: The Viking Press, 1974.

Lesh, T. V. Zen meditation and the Development of Empathy in Counselors. *Journal Human Psychology,* 1970, Vol. 10:39.

Maupin, E. W. Individual Difference in Response to a Zen Meditation Exercise. *Journal of Consulting Psychology,* 1965, Vol. 29 (2): 139-145.

Meares, A. Regression of Cancer After Intensive Meditation. *Medical Journal.* Australia: July 31, 1976, 2:184.

Sanford, J. *Healing and Wholeness.* New York: Paulist Press, 1977.

Schultz, J. H. & Luthe, W. *Autogenic Training.* New York: Grune and Stratton, 1959.

Shafii, M., Lavely R., & Jaffe, R. Meditation and the Prevention of Alcohol Abuse. *American Journal of Psychiatry,* September, 1975, 132:9.

Sperry, R. W. Hemispheric Deconnection and Unity in Conscious Awareness. *American Psychologist.* Vol. 23:10, October, 1968.

Sperry, R. W. The Great Cerebral Commissure. *Scientific American,* January 1964.

Stone, R. A. & DeLeo, J. Psychotherapeutic Control of Hypertension. *The New England Journal of Medicine,* 294:2, January 8, 1976.

Chapter 6

Achterberg, J., Simonton, O. C. & Simonton, S. *Stress, Psychological Factors and Cancer.* Fort Worth: New Medicine Press, 1976.

Bahnson, C. (Ed.). Second Conference on Psychophysiological Aspects of Cancer. *Annals of New York Academy of Sciences,* 1969, Vol. 164, No. 2, 306–634.

Bahnson, C. & Kissen, D. M. (Eds.). Psychophysiological Aspects of Cancer.

Annals of New York Academy of Sciences, 1966, Vol. 125, No. 3, 773–1055.

Bathrop, R. W. Depressed lymphocyte function after bereavement. *Lancet,* April 16, 1977, 834–36.

Benson, H. *Relaxation Response.* New York: William Morrow, 1975.

Homes, T. H. & Rahe, R. H. The Social Readjustment Rating Scale. *Journal of Psychosomatic Research,* 1967, 11, 213–18.

Holmes, T. H. & Masuda, M. *Life Change and Illness Susceptibility.* Paper presented as part of Symposium on Separation and Depression: Clinical and Research Aspects, Chicago, December, 1970.

Hutschnecker, A. A. *The Will To Live.* New York: Thomas Y. Crowell Company, 1953.

Jacobson, E. *Progressive Relaxation* (2nd ed.). Chicago: University of Chicago Press, 1938.

Kissen, D. M. Psychosocial Factors, Personality, and Lung Cancer in Men Aged 55–64. *British Journal of Medical Psychology,* 1967, 40, 29.

LaBarba, R. C. Experimental and Environmental Factors in Cancer. *Psychosomatic Medicine,* 1970, 32, 259.

LeShan, L. L. An Emotional Life History Pattern Associated with Neoplastic Disease. *Annals of the New York Academy of Sciences,* 1966, 125, 780–793.

Riley, V. Mouse Mammary Tumors: Alteration of Incidence as Apparent Function of Stress. *Science,* August, 1975, 189, 465–467.

Ross, E. K. *On Death and Dying.* New York: Macmillan, 1970.

Schmale, A. H. & Iker, H. The Psychological Setting of Uterine Cervical Cancer. *Annals of the New York Academy of Sciences,* 1966, 125, 807–813.

Simonton, O. C. & Simonton, S. Belief Systems and Management of the Emotional Aspects of Malignancy. *Journal of Transpersonal Psychology,* 1975, 7 (1), 29–47.

Simonton, O. C., Simonton, S. M. & Creighton, J. *Getting Well Again.* Los Angeles: J. P. Tarcher, Inc., 1978.

Solomon, G. F. Emotions, Stress, the Central Nervous System and Immunity. *Annals of the New York Academy of Sciences,* 1969, 164, 335–343.

Thomas, C. B. & Duszynski, D. R. Closeness to Parents and the Family Constellation in a Prospective Study of Five Disease States: Suicide,

Mental Illness, Malignant Tumor, Hypertension, and Coronary Heart Disease. *The Johns Hopkins Medical Journal,* 1974, 134, 251-270.

West, P. M., Blumberg, E. M. & Ellis, F. W. An Observed Correlation Between Psychological Factors and Growth Rate of Cancer in Man. *Cancer Research,* 1952, 12, 306-307.

Chapter 7

A Course in Miracles (3 vols.). Foundation for Inner Peace. Box 635E, Tiburon, California: 1975.

Mother Theresa—personal correspondence with the writer (G.G.J.)

Praul, D. Ailing Boy Who Preferred to Die. *San Francisco Chronicle,* January 26, 1978.

Ross, E. K. *On Death and Dying.* New York: Macmillan, 1970.

There is a Rainbow Behind Every Dark Cloud. 19 Main Street, Tiburon, California: Center for Attitudinal Healing, 1978.

Chapter 8

de Chardin, T. *The Phenomenon of Man.* New York: Harper and Row, 1959.

Dickey, L. *Clinical Ecology.* Springfield, Illinois: Charles C. Thomas, 1976.

Feingold, B. *Why Your Child is Hyperactive.* New York: Random House, 1975.

Feldenkrais, M. *Awareness Through Movement.* New York: Harper and Row, 1977.

Harman, D. Prolongation of Life; Role of Free Radical Reactions in Aging. *Journal of American Geriatrics Society,* Vol. 17, No. 8, August 1969, 721-735.

Lowen, A. *Bioenergetics.* New York: Coward, McCann & Geoghegan, 1975.

Maslow, A. *Motivation and Personality.* New York: Harper and Row, 1970.

Ott, J. *Health and Light.* Old Greenwich, Connecticut: Devin-Adair, 1973.

Selye, H. *The Stress of Life.* New York: McGraw-Hill, 1956.

Today's Food and Additives. *General Foods Corp.* White Plains, New York: 1976.

U.S. Environmental Protection Agency. *EPA's Position on the Health Implications of Airborne Lead.* Washington, D.C.: U.S. Government Printing Office, November 28, 1973.

Williams, R. *Biochemical Individuality.* Austin, Texas: University of Texas Press, 1956.

Chapter 9

Bach, M. *The Power of Total Living.* New York: Dodd, Mead & Company, 1977.

Cooper, K. *Aerobics.* Philadelphia: Lippincott, 1968.

de Chardin. T. *The Phenomenon of Man.* New York: Harper & Row, 1959.

Doman, G. *What to Do About Your Brain-Injured Child.* New York: Doubleday & Company, 1974.

Hall, M. P. *Masonic, Hermetic, Cabbalistic, & Rosicrucian Symbolical Philosophy.* Los Angeles: The Philosophical Research Society, Inc., 1977.

Hutschnecker, A. A. *The Will to Live.* New York: Thomas Y. Crowell Co., 1951.

Jayne, W. A. *The Healing Gods of Ancient Civilizations.* New York: University Books, 1962. (Foreword by Thomas E. Gaddis).

Maltz, Maxwell. *Psychocybernetics.* Englewood Cliffs, N.J.: Prentice-Hall, 1960.

Marti-Ibanez, F. *A Prelude to Medical History.* New York: MD Publications, Inc., 1961.

Meier, C. A. *Jung's Analytical Psychology and Religion.* Carbondale, Illinois: Southern Illinois University Press, 1975.

Noss, J. B. *Man's Religions.* New York: The Macmillan Company, 1972.

Oursler, W. *The Healing Power of Faith.* New York: Hawthorn Books, Inc. 1957.

Pruyser, P. W. *A Dynamic Psychology of Religion.* New York: Harper & Row, 1968.

Simeons, A. T. W. *Man's Presumptuous Brain.* New York: E. P. Dutton & Co., 1962.

Szekely, E. B. *The Essene Gospel of Peace.* San Diego, California: Academy Books, 1974.

Tournier, P. *The Whole Person in a Broken World.* New York: Harper & Row, 1965.

Williams & Kalita. *A Physician's Handbook on Orthomolecular Medicine.* Elmsford, N.Y.: Pergamon Press, 1977.

Chapter 10

Belgum, D. (Ed.). *Religion & Medicine.* Ames, Iowa: Iowa State University, 1967.

Clinebell, H. J., Jr. *Basic Types of Pastoral Counseling.* Nashville, Tennessee: Abingdon Press, 1966.

Dicks, R. *Toward Health & Wholeness.* New York: Macmillan Company, 1960.

Frankl, V. *The Doctor & The Soul.* New York: Alfred A. Knopf, 1957.

Fromm, E. *Psychoanalysis & Religion.* New Haven: Yale University Press, 1956.

Holy Bible, The. Revised Standard Version.

Johnson, P. *Psychology of Religion.* Nashville, Tennessee: Abingdon Press, 1959.

Lapsley, N. *Salvation & Health.* Philadelphia: Westminster Press, 1972.

MacNutt, F. *Healing.* Notre Dame, Indiana: Ave Maria Press, 1966.

Menninger, K. *The Vital Balance.* New York: Viking Press, 1963.

Montgomery, D. W. (Ed.). *Healing & Wholeness.* Richmond, Virginia: John Knox Press, 1971.

Oates, W. E. *The Psychology of Religion.* Waco, Texas: Word Books, 1973.

Outler, A. C. *Psychotherapy & The Christian Message.* New York: Harper & Bros., 1954.

Roberts, D. E. *Psychotherapy & A Christian View of Man.* New York: Charles Scribner's Sons, 1950.

Tournier, P. *The Meaning of Persons.* New York: Harper & Bros., 1957.

Young, R. K. & Meiburg, A. L. *Spiritual Therapy.* New York: Harper & Bros., 1960.

Chapter 11

A Course in Miracles (3 Vols.). Box 635E, Tiburon, California: Foundation for Inner Peace, 1975.

Berdyaev, N. *The Destiny of Man.* New York: Harper & Row, 1960, 53–54.

Cliffe, A. E. *Let Go and Let God.* Englewood Cliffs, New Jersey: Prentice-Hall, 1951.

de Saint-Exupery, A. *Wind, Sand and Stars.* New York: Harcourt Brace, 1949.

Eliade, M. *The Sacred and the Profane.* New York: Harcourt Brace, 1949.

Elkes, J. *Education for Health Enhancement.* Presentation at the Annual Meeting of the American Psychiatric Association, Atlanta, Georgia, May 8, 1978.

Frank, J. *Persuasion and Healing.* New York: Shocken Books, 1974.

Frankl, V. *From Death Camp to Existentialism.* Boston: Beacon Press, 1959.

Guggenbühl-Craig, A. *Power in the Helping Professions.* New York: Spring Publications, 1971.

Guirdham, A. *Cosmic Factors in Disease.* London: Duckworth and Co., 1963.

Hayes, D. M. *Between Doctor and Patient.* Valley Forge, Pennsylvania: Judson Press, 1977.

Hillman, J. *Re-Visioning Psychology.* New York: Harper and Row, 1975.

Horton, W. M. *Our Eternal Contemporary.* New York: Harper & Row, 1942, 82–84.

LeShan, L. *How To Meditate.* New York: Bantam Books, 1975.

MacNutt, F. *Healing.* Notre Dame, Indiana: Ave Maria Press, 1974.

Mayeroff, M. *Caring.* New York: Harper & Row, 1971.

Plato. *Charmides.* 155–156/LB15–21.

Psychotherapy: Purpose, Process and Practice. Box 635E, Tiburon, California: Foundation for Inner Peace, 1976.

Wapnick, K. *Christian Psychology in "A Course in Miracles."* Huntington Station, New York: Coleman Graphics, 1978.

Weatherhead, L. D. *Psychology, Religion and Healing.* New York: Abingdon Press, 1952.

Chapter 12

Bean, W. B. (Ed.). *William Osler; Aphorisms from His Bedside Teaching and Writings.* New York: Henry Schuman, Inc., 1950.

Cushing, H. *The Life of Sir William Osler* (2 Vols.). Oxford: Clarendon Press, 1925.

Final Report of the Commission on Medical Education. Office of the Director of Study. New York, 1932.

Flexner, Alexander. *Medical Education in the United States and Canada. A Report to the Carnegie Foundation for the Advancement of Teaching.* Bulletin Number Four (1910). Reproduced in 1960 by Science and Health Publications, Washington, D.C.

MacKenzie, Sir James. *The Future of Medicine.* London: Oxford University Press, 1919.

McDermott, W. Medicine: The Public Good and One's Own. *Perspectives in Biology and Medicine,* 1978, 21:167–187.

Medical Education Since 1960: Marching To a Different Drummer. A Conference of the Kellogg Center for Continuing Education of the Michigan State University, October 18-20, 1978, Lansing, Michigan.

Osler, W. *Whole Time Clinical Professors.* A Letter to President Remsen of Johns Hopkins University. September 1, 1911.

Parke, Davis & Company. *Great Moments in Medicine. A History of Medicine in Pictures.* Detroit: Northwood Institute Press, 1966.

Progress and Problems in Medical and Dental Education; Federal Support Versus Federal Control, A Report of The Carnegie Foundation on Policy Studies in Higher Education. San Francisco, Washington, London: Jossey-Bass, 1976.

Regelson, William. The Weakening of the Oslerian Tradition; The Changing Emphasis in Departments of Medicine. *Journal of the American Medical Association.* 1978, 239:317-319.

The Robert Wood Johnson Foundation Special Report. Number One, 1978. Princeton: The Robert Wood Johnson Foundation.

A Symposium on 6 Year B.S./M.D. Degree Programs. University of Missouri (Kansas City) School of Medicine, December, 1977.

Chapter 13

Belloc, N. B. and Breslow, L. Relationship of Physical Health Status and Health Practices. *Preventive Medicine,* 1972, Vol. 1, pp. 409-421.

Belsky, M. S. & Gross, L. *How to Choose and Use Your Doctor.* New York: Arbor House, 1975.

Boston Women's Health Course Collective: *Our Bodies, Ourselves, A Course By and For Women.* Boston: New England Free Press, 1971.

Burack, R. *The Handbook of Prescription Drugs.* New York: Ballantine Books, 1975.

Cornacchia, H. J. *Consumer Health.* St. Louis: C. V. Mosby, 1976.

Editors of Consumer Reports. *The Medicine Show.* Mt. Vernon, New York: Consumers Union, 1976.

Friedman, M. & Rosenman, R. H. *Type A Behavior and Your Heart.* New York: Fawcett Crest, 1974.

Gaver, J. R. *How to Help Your Doctor Help You.* Los Angeles: Pinnacle Books, Inc., 1975.

Graedon, J. *The People's Pharmacy.* New York: St. Martin's Press, 1976.

Holmes, O. W. In Cornacchia, H. J. *Consumer Health* St. Louis: C. V. Mosby, 1976.

Levin, A. *Talk Back to Your Doctor.* New York: Doubleday, 1975.

Ratner, H. In Mintz, M. *The Therapeutic Nightmare.* Boston: Houghton-Mifflin Co., 1965.

Sehnert, K. W. & Eisenberg, H. *How to Be Your Own Doctor (Sometimes).* New York: Grosset & Dunlap, 1975.

Vickery, D. M. & Fries, J. F. *Take Care of Yourself, A Consumer's Guide to Medical Care.* Reading, Massachusetts: Addison-Wesley, 1976.

Chapter 14

A Course in Miracles (3 Vols.). Box 635E, Tiburon, California: Foundation for Inner Peace, 1975.

Bach, R. *Jonathan Livingston Seagull.* New York: The Macmillan Co., 1970, pp. 76-77.

Becker, R. O. Augmentation of Regenerative Healing in Man: A Possible Alternative to Prosthetic Implantation. *Clinical Orthop.,* March-April, 1972, 83, 255-262.

Becker, R. O. & Spadaro, J. A. Electrical Stimulation of Partial Limb Regeneration in Mammals. *Bulletin New York Academy of Medicine,* May, 1972, 48, 627-641.

Bentov, I. The Mechanics of Consciousness. *New Dimensions of Consciousness Symposium,* November 17-20, 1978, Statler Hilton, New York, N.Y.

Burr, H. S. *Blueprint for Immortality.* London: Neville Spearman, 1972.

Curry, H. Family Practice Perspective. In R. Cunningham and J. Westberg (Eds.). *Report of National Symposium on Wholistic Health Care.* September 15-16, 1977, Hinsdale, Illinois: Wholistic Health Centers.

Daily Word, Unity Village, Missouri: Unity School of Christianity.

Dean, S. R. *Psychiatry and Mysticism.* Chicago, Illinois: Nelson Hall, 1975.

Jason, H. Developing the Providers. In R. Cunningham and J. Westberg (Eds.). *Report of National Symposium on Wholistic Health Care.* September 15-16, 1977, Hinsdale, Illinois: Wholistic Health Centers.

Lily, J. C. *The Deep Self.* New York: Simon & Schuster, 1977.

Maloney, W. F. A Physician's Reaction. In R. Cunningham and J. Westberg (Eds.). *Report of National Symposium on Wholistic Health Care.* September 15-16, 1977, Hinsdale, Illinois: Wholistic Health Centers.

Pribram, K. New Directions in the Scientific Explorations of Consciousness, *New Dimensions of Consciousness Symposium,* November 17-20, 1978, Statler Hilton, New York, N.Y.

Progoff, I. *ATA Journal Workshop.* New York: Dialogue House Library, 1975.

Toffler, A. *Future Shock.* New York: Random House, Inc., 1970.

Weil, A. *The Natural Mind.* Boston, Massachusetts: Houghton Mifflin Co., 1972.

Smith, J. Bioenergetics in Healing. In R. Carlson (Ed.). *The Frontiers of Science and Medicine,* Chicago: Henry Regnery Co., 1975.

Epilogue

Bach, S. R. von. Spontanes Malen Schwerkanker Patienten. *Arta Psychosomatica.* Basle, Switzerland, 1966.

Ross, E. E. *Coping with Death and Dying: A Set of Teaching Tapes.* 1825 Sylvan Court, Flossmoor, Ill., Ross Medical Associates.

Ross, E. K. *On Death and Dying.* New York: Macmillian Publishing Company, Inc., 1969.

Ross, E. K. *Questions and Answers on Death and Dying.* New York: Macmillian Publishing Company, Inc., 1974.

Ross, E. K. *Death, the Final Stage of Growth.* Englewood Cliffs: Prentice-Hall, Inc., 1975.

Ross, E. K. *To Live Until We Say Goodbye.* Englewood Cliffs: Prentice-Hall, Inc., 1978.

Additional Reading

Appley, M. H. & Trumbull, R. (Eds.) *Psychological Stress.* New York: Appleton-Century-Crofts, 1967.

Bailes, F. *Your Mind Can Heal You.* Santa Monica, California: Devorss & Co., 1971.

Balint, M. *The Doctor, His Patient & The Illness* (2nd ed.). London: Pitman Medical Publishing, 1964.

Bayly, M. B. The Basic Principles of Health and Disease. *Medical World,* July 6, 1934, 519-524.

Basowitz, H., Persky, H. Korchin, S. J., & Grinker, R. R. *Anxiety and Stress.* New York: McGraw-Hill, 1955.

Beisser, R. Denial and Affirmation in Illness and Health. *Department of Psychiatry,* 1977, University of California, Los Angeles.

Benson, H. & Epstein, M. D. The Placebo Effect: A Neglected Asset in the Care of Patients. *JAMA,* 1975, Vol. 232, No. 12.

Benson, H. *The Relaxation Response.* New York: Morrow, 1975.

Beorse, B. In Search of Mystic Balance. *New Age,* March, 1978.

Bergen, S. S., Jr. The Crisis in Access. *Archives Internal Medicine,* 1976, 136, 721-724.

Bernard, C. *An Introduction to the Study of Experimental Medicine.* New York: Macmillan, 1927.

Bernard, J. *A Doctor Diagnoses the Medical Revolution.* New York: Macmillan, 1975.

Bloomfield, H. H. & Kory, R. B. *Health & Happiness.* New York: Simon & Schuster, 1978.

Bronowski, J. *A Sense of the Future.* Cambridge, Mass: MIT Press, 1977.

Burr, H. S. *Blueprint for Immortality.* London: Neville Spearman, 1972.

Carlson, R. J. (Ed.). *The Frontiers of Science and Medicine.* Chicago: Henry Regnery Co., 1975.

Carlson, R. J. *The End of Medicine.* New York: John Wiley & Sons, 1975.

Carrel, A. *Man The Unknown.* New York: Harper & Bros., 1935.

Cheraskin, E. The Name of the Game is the Name. *Proceedings of the San Diego Biomedical Symposium,* 1974, 13.

Cheraskin, E. & Ringsdorf, W. M. *Predictive Medicine.* Mountain View, CA: Pacific Press, 1973.

A Course in Miracles (3 Vols.). Box 635E, Tiburon, California: Foundation for Inner Peace, 1975.

Cousins, N. What I Learned from 3000 Doctors. *Saturday Review,* Feb. 18, 1978.

Cousins, N. *The Celebration of Life.* New York; Harper & Row, 1974.

Cunningham, R., Jr., & Westberg, J. (Eds.). *Report—National Symposium on Wholistic Health Care,* Sept, 15-16, 1977. Hinsdale, Ill: Wholistic Health Centers, 1977.

Dean, R. *Psychiatry and Mysticism.* Chicago: Nelson Hall, 1975.

The Dimensions of Healing: A Symposium. Los Angeles: Academy of Parapsychology and Medicine, 1972.

Dubos, Rene. *The Mirage of Health.* New York: Harper & Bros., 1959.

Edmunds, H., and Associates. *Some Unrecognized Factors in Medicine.* Wheaton, Ill.: Theosophical Publishing House, 1976.

Elgin, D. The Ethics of Psi. *New Age,* March, 1978.

Engel, L. Homeostasis, Behavioral Adjustment, and the Concept of Health and Disease. In R. Grinker (Ed.), *Mid-Century Psychiatry,* Springfield, Ill.: Charles C. Thomas, 1953.

Engel, G. L. The Need for a New Medical Model: A Challenge for Biomedicine. *Science,* 1977, 196, 129-136.

Engel, G. L. *Psychological Development in Health and Disease.* Philadelphia: W. B. Saunders Co., 1962.

Evans, I. *Carl Rogers: The Man and His Ideas.* New York: E. P. Dutton, 1975.

Frank, J. D. *Persuasion and Healing.* Baltimore: Johns Hopkins University Press, 1973.

Frankl, V. E. *The Doctor and the Soul.: From Psychotherapy to Logotherapy.* New York: Alfred Knopf, 1965.

Frankl, V. E. *Man's Search for Meaning.* New York: Pocket Books, 1959.

Frankl, V. E. *The Unconscious God: Psychotherapy and Theology.* New York: Simon & Schuster, 1976.

Galdston, I. *The Meaning of Social Medicine.* Cambridge, Mass.: Harvard University Press, 1954.

Gardner, J. W. *No Easy Victories.* New York: Harper & Row, 1968.

Glasser, R. J. *The Body is the Hero.* New York: Random House, 1976.

Goldberg, P. & Kaufman, D. *Natural Sleep.* Emmaus, PA: Rodale Press, 1978.

Grace, W. J. & Graham, D. T. The Specificity of the Relation between Attitudes and Disease. *Psychosomatic Medicine,* 1952, 14:243 No. 4.

Green, E. & Green, A. *Beyond Biofeedback.* New York: Delta, 1977.

Grinker, R. *Mid-Century Psychiatry.* Springfield, Illinois: Charles C. Thomas, 1953.

Hall, R. H. Counter-effects of Medical Technology. *Journal of the International Society for Technology Assessment,* March, 1975, 29-36.

Halstead, L. S. & Halstead, M. G. Chronic Illness and Humanism. *Reha-*

bilitation as a Model for Teaching Humanistic Health Care. *Archives of Physical Medicine and Rehabilitation,* 1978, 59, 53–57.

Hayes, D. M. *Between Doctor and Patient.* Valley Forge, Pennsylvania: Judson Press, 1977.

Jacobson, E. *You Must Relax.* New York: McGraw-Hill Book Co., 1957.

Joy, B. *Joy's Way.* Los Angeles: J. P. Tarcher, 1979.

Jung, C. G. *The Undiscovered Self.* Boston: Little, Brown & Co., 1957.

Koestler, A. *The Roots of Coincidence.* New York: Vintage Books, 1973.

Knowles, J. H. (Ed.). *Doing Better and Feeling Worse.* New York: W. W. Norton & Co., 1977.

Knowles, J. Responsibility for Health. *Science,* 1977, 198.

Knowles, J. H. (Ed.). *Views of Medical Education and Medical Care.* Cambridge, Massachusetts: Harvard University Press, 1968.

Krauklis, A. A. *Self Regulation of Higher Nervous Activity.* January 22, 1964. Academy of Sciences of the Latvian SSR.

Lazarus, R. S. *Psychological Stress and the Coping Process.* New York: McGraw-Hill, 1966.

Meek, W. (Ed.). *Healers and the Healing Process.* Wheaton, Illinois: The Theosophical Publishing House, 1977.

Miller, S., Remen, N., Barbour, A., Miller, S. & Garrell, D. *Dimensions of Humanistic Medicine.* San Francisco: Institute for the Study of Humanistic Medicine, 1975.

Noble, C. P. The Prevention and Cure of What is Called Old Age—Premature Senescence. *Medical World,* July, 1934; 367–370.

Ornstein, R. E. *The Psychology of Consciousness.* San Francisco: W. H. Freeman and Co., 1972.

Oyle, I. *The Healing Mind.* Millbrae, California: Celestial Arts, 1975.

Palmer, R. E. The AMA's Health Plan. *Newsweek,* June 6, 1977, 11–12.

Pelletier, K. R. *Mind as Healer, Mind as Slayer.* New York: Delta, 1977.

Progoff, I. *The Cloud of Unknowing.* New York: Delta, 1957.

Progoff, I. *ATA Journal Workshop.* New York: Dialogue House Library, 1975.

Rahe, R. H. & Arthur, R. J. Life Change and Illness Studies: Past History and Future Directions. *Journal of Human Stress,* March, 1978.

Sanford, J. A. *Healing and Wholeness.* New York: Paulist Press, 1966.

Seelig, C. (Ed.). *Ideas and Opinions by Albert Einstein.* New York: Crown Publishers, 1954.

Selye, H. *In Vivo: The Case for Supramolecular Biology.* New York: Liveright Publishing Corp., 1967.

Selye, H. *Stress Without Distress.* Philadelphia: J. B. Lippincott Company, 1974.

Selye, H. *The Stress of Life* (Rev. ed.). New York: McGraw-Hill, 1976.

Shealy, C. N. *90 Days to Self Health.* New York: The Dial Press, 1977.

Smith, A. *Powers of the Mind.* New York: Random House, 1975.

Snively, W. D., Jr. & Thuerbach, J. *Healing Beyond Medicine.* West Nyack, New Jersey: Parker Publishing Co., 1972.

Swaim, L. T. *Arthritis, Medicine and the Spiritual Laws.* Philadelphia: Chilton Book Co., 1962.

Thetford, W. N. & Schucman, H. Motivational Factors and Adaptive Behavior. *Physiological Basis of Rehabilitation Medicine.* Darling & Downey; Williams & Wilkins.

Totman, R. *Social Causes of Illness.* London: Souvenir Press, Ltd., 1979.

Index